PROCEDURE CHECKLISTS

to Accompany

NURSING FUNDAMENTALS

CARING & CLINICAL DECISION MAKING

Rick Daniels

Prepared by

Lisa J. Oswalt, RN, MSN, BC
Instructor in Nursing
School of Nursing
Delta State University
Cleveland, Mississippi

Karrin Johnson, RN
Health Care Project Manager
NRSPACE Software, Inc.
Bellevue, Washington

DELMAR

™

THOMSON LEARNING

Australia Canada Mexico Singapore Spain United Kingdom United States

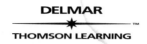

Procedure Checklists to Accompany
Nursing Fundamentals: Caring & Clinical Decision Making

by Rick Daniels

prepared by Lisa Oswalt and Karrin Johnson

VP of Healthcare SBU:
William Brottmiller

Editorial Director:
Cathy L. Esperti

Acquisitions Editor:
Matthew Filimonov

Senior Developmental Editor:
Elisabeth F. Williams

Marketing Director:
Jennifer McAvey

Channel Manager:
Tamara Caruso

Project Editor:
Mary Ellen Cox

Editorial Assistant:
Patricia M. Osborn

Art/Design Coordinator:
Connie Lundberg-Watkins

Production Coordinator:
Kenneth McGrath

Library of Congress Cataloging-in-Publication Data

ISBN: 1-4018-4045-0

INTERNATIONAL DIVISIONS LIST

Asia (including India):
Thomson Learning
60 Albert Street, #15-01
Albert Complex
Singapore 189969
Tel 65 336-6411
Fax 65 336-7411

Australia/New Zealand:
Nelson
102 Dodds Street
South Melbourne
Victoria 3205
Australia
Tel 61 (0)3 9685-4111
Fax 61 (0)3 9685-4111

Latin America:
Thomson Learning
Seneca 53
Colonia Polanco
11560 Mexico, D.F. Mexico
Tel (525) 281-2906
Fax (525) 2656

Canada:
Nelson
1120 Birchmount Road
Toronto, Ontario
Canada M1K 5G4
Tel (416) 752-9100
Fax (416) 8102

UK/Europe/Middle East/Africa:
Thomson Learning
Berkshire House
1680-173 High Holborn
London WC1V 7AA
United Kingdom
Tel 44 (0)20 497-1422
Fax 44 (0)20 497-1426

Spain (includes Portugal):
Paraninfo
Calle Megallanes 25
28015 Madrid
España
Tel 34 (0)91 446-3350
Fax 34 (0)91 445-6218

NOTICE TO THE READER

CONTENTS

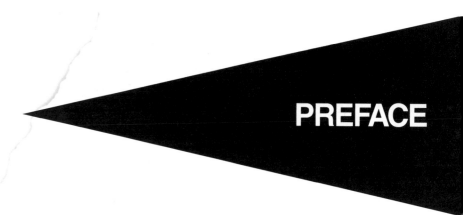

PREFACE

The procedure checklists in this manual are summaries of the step-by-step procedures in *Nursing Fundamentals: Caring & Clinical Decision Making*. These checklists are numbered to correspond to the procedure numbers in the main textbook. The checklists are designed to facilitate evaluation of a student's performance of the first three steps of the nursing process related to each skill:

- Assessment
- Planning/Expected Outcomes
- Implementation

The steps in each checklist follow the steps of the procedure as described in the textbook. To use the checklists more effectively, the student should refer to the procedure in the textbook first, then "practice" the skill referring to the checklist.

When students are evaluated using the checklists, there are three categories to document their performance of the skills: "Able to Perform," "Able to Perform with Assistance," or "Unable to Perform." These categories lend themselves to the college laboratory setting as well as to the clinical setting, where students may perform procedures with faculty assistance.

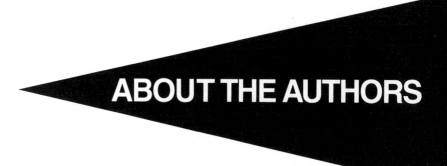

ABOUT THE AUTHORS

Lisa J. Oswalt, RN, MSN, BC, is a nursing instructor at Delta State University School of Nursing in Cleveland, Mississippi. She has been on the faculty at this university for 9 years, with teaching assignments in pediatrics, fundamentals, nursing management, and writing for professional nursing. She is an ANCC Board Certified Pediatric Nurse and continues to practice nursing in her hometown. During her 15 years as a registered nurse she has worked in various roles, including medical-surgical, cardiac step-down, pediatrics, and education coordinator. She is a charter member of the Pi Xi Chapter of Sigma Theta Tau International and the National League for Nursing, and is active in a variety of university, professional, and community service activities. She lives in Cleveland with her husband, Danny, and son, Dean.

Karrin Johnson, RN, is currently working with the staff at NRSPACE Software to develop educational texts and software for the health care industry. She has worked as a nurse for twenty years, spending much of that time in the intensive care and coronary care settings. She currently lives in Seattle, Washington, with her sons, Aaron and Timothy.

Checklist for Procedure 26-1　Handwashing

Name _____ Date _____

School _____

Instructor _____

Course _____

Procedure 26-1 Handwashing	Able to Perform	Able to Perform with Assistance	Unable to Perform	Initials and Date
Assessment				
1. Assess the environment. *Comments:*	☐	☐	☐	
2. Assess your hands. *Comments:*	☐	☐	☐	
Planning/Expected Outcomes				
1. The caregiver's hands will be cleansed adequately to remove microorganisms, transient flora, and soil from the skin. *Comments:*	☐	☐	☐	
Implementation				
1. Remove jewelry. Push sleeves of uniform or shirt up. *Comments:*	☐	☐	☐	
2. Assess hands for hangnails, cuts or breaks in the skin, and areas that are heavily soiled. *Comments:*	☐	☐	☐	
3. Turn on the water. Adjust the flow and temperature. *Comments:*	☐	☐	☐	
4. Wet hands and lower forearms thoroughly by holding under warm running water. Keep hands and forearms in the down position with elbows straight. *Comments:*	☐	☐	☐	
5. Apply about 5 ml (1 teaspoon) of liquid soap. Lather thoroughly. *Comments:*	☐	☐	☐	

　　　　continued on the following page

continued from the previous page

Procedure 26-1	Able to Perform	Able to Perform with Assistance	Unable to Perform	Initials and Date
6. Thoroughly rub hands together for about 10 to 15 seconds. *Comments:*	☐	☐	☐	
7. Rinse with hands in the down position, elbows straight. Rinse in the direction of forearm to wrist to fingers. *Comments:*	☐	☐	☐	
8. Blot hands and forearms to dry thoroughly. Dry in the direction of fingers to wrist and forearms. Discard the paper towels in the proper receptacle. *Comments:*	☐	☐	☐	
9. Turn off the water faucet with a clean, dry paper towel. *Comments:*	☐	☐	☐	

_____   _____

Faculty Signature   Date

Checklist for Procedure 26-2   Surgical Asepsis: Preparing and Maintaining a Sterile Field

Name _____ Date _____

School _____

Instructor _____

Course _____

Procedure 26-2 Surgical Asepsis: Preparing and Maintaining a Sterile Field	Able to Perform	Able to Perform with Assistance	Unable to Perform	Initials and Date
Assessment				
1. Assess the environment. *Comments:*	☐	☐	☐	
2. Assess the client for situation that requires preparation of a sterile field. *Comments:*	☐	☐	☐	
Planning/Expected Outcomes				
1. The client will have no nosocomial infection or related opportunistic infections as a result of improper preparation or maintenance of a sterile field. *Comments:*	☐	☐	☐	
Implementation				
1. Gather equipment and supplies specific for the type of procedure. *Comments:*	☐	☐	☐	
2. Obtain only intact, clean, and dry packages marked "sterile." *Comments:*	☐	☐	☐	
3. Check all packages for expiration date and integrity. *Comments:*	☐	☐	☐	
4. Locate a clean, dry, flat surface in the client's environment on which to prepare the sterile field. *Comments:*	☐	☐	☐	
5. Explain the procedure to the client. *Comments:*	☐	☐	☐	

continued on the following page

continued from the previous page

Procedure 26-2	Able to Perform	Able to Perform with Assistance	Unable to Perform	Initials and Date
6. Provide additional instruction as indicated for specific procedures or testing that require a sterile field. *Comments:*	☐	☐	☐	
7. If the client is in a private room, close the door to maintain privacy. If the client is not in a private room, move the client to an exam room if possible or provide for privacy. *Comments:*	☐	☐	☐	
8. Position the client in a comfortable position that will allow accessibility of the area. The bed position should facilitate proper body mechanics. *Comments:*	☐	☐	☐	
9. Wash hands. *Comments:*	☐	☐	☐	
10. Place sterile package in the center of a clean, dry surface at waist height (if possible). *Comments:*	☐	☐	☐	
11. Remove the wrapper (if indicated), pulling the wrapper away from the body. *Comments:*	☐	☐	☐	
12. Grasp the folded top edge of the inner paper cover with fingertips of one hand. *Comments:*	☐	☐	☐	
13. Remove the drape by lifting up and away from objects as it unfolds. *Comments:*	☐	☐	☐	
14. With free hand, grasp the other corner of the lower drape and pull toward you, being careful not to touch inner contents. *Comments:*	☐	☐	☐	
15. Lay the tray on the work surface so that the top flap of the sterile wrapper is away from you. *Comments:*	☐	☐	☐	

Procedure 26-2	Able to Perform	Able to Perform with Assistance	Unable to Perform	Initials and Date
16. Reach around the tray with the thumb and index finger, and grasp the wrapper's top flap. Gently pull the flap up, then down to open over the work surface. *Comments:*	☐	☐	☐	
17. Repeat step 16 to open all remaining flaps. *Comments:*	☐	☐	☐	
18. Grasp the corner of the bottom flap with the fingertips, step back, and pull the flap down. *Comments:*	☐	☐	☐	
19. While facing the sterile field, step back and remove the outer wrapper, and grasp the item in your nondominant hand so that the top flap will open away from you. *Comments:*	☐	☐	☐	
20. With your dominant hand, open the flaps as in step 16 and repeat the process for each flap. *Comments:*	☐	☐	☐	
21. With your dominant hand, pull the wrapper back and away from the sterile field and place the item in the sterile field. *Comments:*	☐	☐	☐	
22. When adding additional gauze or dressings to the sterile field, open the packages as directed, grasp the top of the packaging and gently pull the wrapper downward. Then drop the contents onto the sterile field. *Comments:*	☐	☐	☐	
23. When adding solutions to the sterile field, read all labels three (3) times before pouring. *Comments:*	☐	☐	☐	
24. Remove the lid from the solution and place on the surface with the cap opening facing up. *Comments:*	☐	☐	☐	

continued on the following page

continued from the previous page

Procedure 26-2	Able to Perform	Able to Perform with Assistance	Unable to Perform	Initials and Date
25. Hold the bottle with the label facing the palm of the hand, 4 to 5 inches over the sterile container to be used in the sterile field. *Comments:*	☐	☐	☐	
26. Pour the solution slowly and without touching the container. *Comments:*	☐	☐	☐	
27. Replace the lid on the container, and label the container with your initials, the date, and the time if retained for future use. *Comments:*	☐	☐	☐	
28. Wash hands *Comments:*	☐	☐	☐	
29. Don nonsterile gloves *Comments:*	☐	☐	☐	
30. With dominant hand, grasp forceps from the sterile field, making sure to touch only the handles. *Comments:*	☐	☐	☐	
31. Hold the forceps above waist level at all times during the procedure. *Comments:*	☐	☐	☐	
32. Keep forceps tips positioned downward when adding, arranging, or removing items to the sterile field during the procedure. *Comments:*	☐	☐	☐	
33. Dispose of contaminated supplies and replace if indicated, using sterile techniques discussed. *Comments:*	☐	☐	☐	
34. Wash hands. *Comments:*	☐	☐	☐	

Procedure 26-2	Able to Perform	Able to Perform with Assistance	Unable to Perform	Initials and Date
35. Don sterile gloves using open gloving technique (Procedure 26-3). *Comments:*	☐	☐	☐	
36. Continue with the procedure, keeping gloved hands above the waist and in view at all times during the procedure. *Comments:*	☐	☐	☐	
37. If using a solution for cleansing, use the sterile forceps to prevent contamination of gloves. Dispose of forceps after use. *Comments:*	☐	☐	☐	
38. Post-procedure: Dispose of all contaminated items in biohazard materials bags. Dispose of trash in appropriate receptacle. *Comments:*	☐	☐	☐	
39. Remove gloves by grasping the outside of one glove cuff with the other gloved hand; pull the glove off turning it inside out. Curl this glove in a ball in the gloved hand. Take the index finger from the ungloved hand and place the index finger underneath the inner cuff area (at the wrist) of the glove. Use a downward pulling motion. *Comments:*	☐	☐	☐	
40. Wash hands. *Comments:*	☐	☐	☐	
41. Reposition the client and ensure client's safety. *Comments:*	☐	☐	☐	
42. Clean the environment. *Comments:*	☐	☐	☐	
43. Document procedure. *Comments:*	☐	☐	☐	

Faculty Signature　　　　　　　　　　　　　　　　　　　　Date

　　　continued on the following page

Checklist for Procedure 26-3　Applying Sterile Gloves via the Open Method

Name _____ Date _____

School _____

Instructor _____

Course _____

Procedure 26-3 Applying Sterile Gloves via the Open Method	Able to Perform	Able to Perform with Assistance	Unable to Perform	Initials and Date
Assessment				
1.　Assess the glove package. 　　*Comments:*	☐	☐	☐	
2.　Assess the local environment. 　　*Comments:*	☐	☐	☐	
Planning/Expected Outcomes				
1.　Sterility of the gloves will be maintained while they are 　　being applied. 　　*Comments:*	☐	☐	☐	
2.　Sterility of the procedure will be maintained. 　　*Comments:*	☐	☐	☐	
Implementation				
1.　Wash hands. 　　*Comments:*	☐	☐	☐	
2.　Remove the outer wrapper from the package. Place the 　　inner wrapper onto a clean, dry surface. Surface should be 　　at or above waist-height level. Open inner wrapper to 　　expose gloves. 　　*Comments:*	☐	☐	☐	
3.　Identify right and left hand; glove dominant hand first. 　　*Comments:*	☐	☐	☐	
4.　Grasp the 2-inch (5-cm)-wide cuff with the thumb and first 　　two fingers of the nondominant hand, touching only the 　　cuff. 　　*Comments:*	☐	☐	☐	

　　　　continued on the following page

continued from the previous page

Procedure 26-3	Able to Perform	Able to Perform with Assistance	Unable to Perform	Initials and Date
5. Gently pull the glove over the dominant hand. Hold hands above the waist while applying glove. Once dominant hand is gloved, keep hands visible and above waist to prevent accidental contamination. *Comments:*	☐	☐	☐	
6. With the gloved dominant hand, slip your fingers under the cuff of the other glove. *Comments:*	☐	☐	☐	
7. Gently slip the glove onto nondominant hand. Be careful not to drag glove or touch gloved dominant hand with ungloved nondominant hand. *Comments:*	☐	☐	☐	
8. With gloved hands, interlock fingers to fit the gloves onto each finger. *Comments:*	☐	☐	☐	
9. If the gloves are soiled, remove as follows: Slip gloved fingers of the dominant hand under the cuff of the opposite hand, or grasp the outer part of the glove at the wrist if there is no cuff. *Comments:*	☐	☐	☐	
10. Pull the glove down to the fingers, exposing the thumb. *Comments:*	☐	☐	☐	
11. Slip the uncovered thumb into the opposite glove at the wrist. *Comments:*	☐	☐	☐	
12. Pull the glove down over the dominant hand almost to the fingertips and slip the glove onto the other hand. *Comments:*	☐	☐	☐	
13. Pull the glove over the dominant hand so that only the inside is exposed. *Comments:*	☐	☐	☐	
14. Dispose of soiled gloves and wash hands. *Comments:*	☐	☐	☐	

_____   _____
Faculty Signature   Date

Checklist for Procedure 26-4   Donning a Cap and Mask

Name _____ Date _____

School _____

Instructor _____

Course _____

Procedure 26-4 Donning a Cap and Mask	Able to Perform	Able to Perform with Assistance	Unable to Perform	Initials and Date
Assessment				
1. Assess the specific isolation precautions needed for the client's condition. *Comments:*	☐	☐	☐	
2. Assess the client's laboratory results. *Comments:*	☐	☐	☐	
3. Assess what nursing measures are required before entering the room. *Comments:*	☐	☐	☐	
4. Assess the client's knowledge for the need to wear a cap and mask during care. *Comments:*	☐	☐	☐	
5. Assess the type of surgical procedure being done. *Comments:*	☐	☐	☐	
Planning/Expected Outcomes				
1. The client will interact on a social level with the nurse, family members, and other visitors. *Comments:*	☐	☐	☐	
2. The client will remain free of a nosocomial infection. *Comments:*	☐	☐	☐	
3. The staff will be protected from infection when caring for the client. *Comments:*	☐	☐	☐	
4. The staff will avoid transmitting microorganisms to others. *Comments:*	☐	☐	☐	

continued on the following page

continued from the previous page

Procedure 26-4	Able to Perform	Able to Perform with Assistance	Unable to Perform	Initials and Date
Implementation				
1. Wash hands. *Comments:*	☐	☐	☐	
2. Apply cap to head, being sure to tuck hair under cap. Males with facial hair should use a hood to cover all hair on head and face. *Comments:*	☐	☐	☐	
3. Secure mask around mouth and nose. *Comments:*	☐	☐	☐	
4. Enter the client's room and explain the rationale for wearing a cap and mask. *Comments:*	☐	☐	☐	
5. After performing necessary tasks, remove cap and mask before leaving room. *Comments:*	☐	☐	☐	

Faculty Signature

Date

Checklist for Procedure 26-5   Surgical Scrub

Name _____ Date _____

School _____

Instructor _____

Course _____

Procedure 26-5 Surgical Scrub	Able to Perform	Able to Perform with Assistance	Unable to Perform	Initials and Date
Assessment				
1. Assess the scrub environment for equipment and cleanliness. *Comments:*	☐	☐	☐	
2. Assess your preparedness. *Comments:*	☐	☐	☐	
Planning/Expected Outcomes				
1. Hands and forearms will be adequately cleansed for applying sterile gloves and gown. *Comments:*	☐	☐	☐	
Implementation				
Preparation				
1. Remove jewelry and chipped nail polish. *Comments:*	☐	☐	☐	
2. Use a deep sink with side or foot pedal to dispense soap and control water flow. *Comments:*	☐	☐	☐	
3. Have two surgical scrub brushes and nail file available. *Comments:*	☐	☐	☐	
4. Apply surgical shoe covers and cap. *Comments:*	☐	☐	☐	
5. Apply mask. *Comments:*	☐	☐	☐	

                  continued on the following page

continued from the previous page

Procedure 26-5	Able to Perform	Able to Perform with Assistance	Unable to Perform	Initials and Date
6a. Open the sterile package containing the gown and form a sterile field. *Comments:*	☐	☐	☐	
6b. Open the sterile towel and drop it onto the center of field. *Comments:*	☐	☐	☐	
6c. Open the sterile gloves and drop the inner package of gloves onto the sterile field. *Comments:*	☐	☐	☐	
Surgical Handwashing 7. At the sink, under warm flowing water, wet forearms and hands. *Comments:*	☐	☐	☐	
8. Apply soap and rub hands and arms to 2 inches above elbows. *Comments:*	☐	☐	☐	
9. Clean under each nail of both hands and drop file into sink. *Comments:*	☐	☐	☐	
10. With soapy scrub brush in your dominant hand using a circular motion, scrub nails and all skin areas of nondominant hand and arm. *Comments:*	☐	☐	☐	
11. Rinse brush thoroughly; reapply soap. *Comments:*	☐	☐	☐	
12. Continue with scrub of nondominant arm. Drop brush into the sink. *Comments:*	☐	☐	☐	
13. Rinse nondominant fingers, hand, and arm. *Comments:*	☐	☐	☐	

Procedure 26-5	Able to Perform	Able to Perform with Assistance	Unable to Perform	Initials and Date
14. With the second scrub brush, repeat steps 10 through 13 on your dominant hand and arm. *Comments:*	☐	☐	☐	
15. Keep arms flexed and proceed to area with sterile field. *Comments:*	☐	☐	☐	
16. Grasp the sterile towel on one edge, allowing it to fall open. *Comments:*	☐	☐	☐	
17. Dry each hand and arm separately with a rotating motion up to the elbow. *Comments:*	☐	☐	☐	
18. Thoroughly dry the skin. *Comments:*	☐	☐	☐	
19. Discard the towel into a linen hamper. *Comments:*	☐	☐	☐	

Faculty Signature   Date

Checklist for Procedure 26-6　Applying Sterile Gloves and Gown via the Closed Method

Name _____ Date _____

School _____

Instructor _____

Course _____

Procedure 26-6 **Applying Sterile Gloves and Gown** **via the Closed Method**	Able to Perform	Able to Perform with Assistance	Unable to Perform	Initials and Date
Assessment				
1. Assess the surrounding environment. *Comments:*	☐	☐	☐	
2. Assess the condition of your hands. *Comments:*	☐	☐	☐	
Planning/Expected Outcomes				
1. The caregiver will don a sterile gown and gloves without compromising their sterility. *Comments:*	☐	☐	☐	
Implementation				
Gowning 1. The sterile gown comes folded inside out. *Comments:*	☐	☐	☐	
2. Grasp the gown inside the neckline, step back, and allow it to fall open. *Comments:*	☐	☐	☐	
3. Slip both arms into the gown; keep your hands inside the sleeves of the gown. *Comments:*	☐	☐	☐	
4. The circulating nurse will secure the ties at the neck and waist. *Comments:*	☐	☐	☐	
Closed Gloving 5. With hands still inside the gown sleeves, open the inner wrapper of the sterile gloves. *Comments:*	☐	☐	☐	

　　　　　continued on the following page

continued from the previous page

Procedure 26-6	Able to Perform	Able to Perform with Assistance	Unable to Perform	Initials and Date
6. With your nondominant sleeved hand, place the palm of the dominant-hand glove against the sleeved palm of the dominant hand. *Comments:*	☐	☐	☐	
7. Grasp the glove cuff with your dominant, sleeved thumb. With your nondominant hand, turn the cuff over the end of dominant hand and gown's cuff. *Comments:*	☐	☐	☐	
8. While holding the glove and gown cuffs securely, slowly extend the fingers into the glove. *Comments:*	☐	☐	☐	
9. With the gloved dominant hand, repeat steps 7 and 8. *Comments:*	☐	☐	☐	
10. Interlock gloved fingers and secure fit. *Comments:*	☐	☐	☐	

_____

Faculty Signature

_____

Date

Checklist for Procedure 27-1   Taking a Temperature

Name _____ Date _____

School _____

Instructor _____

Course _____

Procedure 27-1 Taking a Temperature	Able to Perform	Able to Perform with Assistance	Unable to Perform	Initials and Date
Assessment				
1. Assess body temperature for changes due to exposure to pyrogens or to extreme hot or cold external environments. *Comments:*	☐	☐	☐	
2. Assess the client for the most appropriate site to check his temperature. *Comments:*	☐	☐	☐	
3. Confirm that the client has not consumed hot or cold foods nor smoked just before the measurement of an oral temperature. *Comments:*	☐	☐	☐	
4. Assess for mouth breathing and tachypnea. *Comments:*	☐	☐	☐	
5. Assess for oral herpetic lesions. *Comments:*	☐	☐	☐	
Planning/Expected Outcomes				
1. An accurate temperature reading will be obtained. *Comments:*	☐	☐	☐	
2. The client will verbalize understanding of the reason for the procedure. *Comments:*	☐	☐	☐	
Implementation				
Preparation 1. Review medical record for factors that influence vital signs. *Comments:*	☐	☐	☐	

                    continued on the following page

continued from the previous page

Procedure 27-1	Able to Perform	Able to Perform with Assistance	Unable to Perform	Initials and Date
2. Explain to the client that vital signs will be assessed. *Comments:*	☐	☐	☐	
3. Assess client's toileting needs and proceed as appropriate. *Comments:*	☐	☐	☐	
4. Gather equipment as indicated above. *Comments:*	☐	☐	☐	
5. Provide for privacy. *Comments:*	☐	☐	☐	
6. Wash hands and apply gloves. *Comments:*	☐	☐	☐	
7. Position the client in a sitting or lying position with the head of the bed elevated 45°–60°, unless taking a rectal or tympanic temperature. *Comments:*	☐	☐	☐	
8. Wash hands when finished performing skill. *Comments:*	☐	☐	☐	
Oral Temperature: Glass Thermometer 9. Select correct thermometer from client's bedside container. Note: Color tip indicates type of thermometer: blue = oral; red = rectal. Bulb indicates type of thermometer: elongated bulb = oral; blunt, rounded bulb = rectal. *Comments:*	☐	☐	☐	
10. Remove thermometer from storage container and cleanse under cool water. *Comments:*	☐	☐	☐	
11. Use a tissue to dry thermometer from the bulb toward fingertips. *Comments:*	☐	☐	☐	
12. Read thermometer by locating mercury level. It should read 35.5°C (96°F). *Comments:*	☐	☐	☐	

Procedure 27-1	Able to Perform	Able to Perform with Assistance	Unable to Perform	Initials and Date
13. If mercury level is not below 96° F, grasp thermometer firmly with thumb and index finger and shake with fluid, wrist-jerking movements. *Comments:*	☐	☐	☐	
14. Place thermometer in client's mouth under the tongue and along the gumline. Instruct client to hold lips closed. *Comments:*	☐	☐	☐	
15. Leave in place 3 to 5 minutes. *Comments:*	☐	☐	☐	
16. Have client open mouth. Remove thermometer. Remove excess secretions, if indicated, with a tissue, wiping from finger tips to bulb. *Comments:*	☐	☐	☐	
17. Read at eye level, rotating slowly until mercury level is visualized. *Comments:*	☐	☐	☐	
18. Record reading and indicate site as "oral." *Comments:*	☐	☐	☐	
19. Shake thermometer down, cleanse, rinse, and return to storage. *Comments:*	☐	☐	☐	
20. Remove and dispose of gloves in appropriate receptacle. *Comments:*	☐	☐	☐	
21. Wash hands. *Comments:*	☐	☐	☐	
Oral Temperature: Electronic Thermometer 22. Repeat steps 1 through 8. *Comments:*	☐	☐	☐	
23. Place disposable protective sheath over probe. *Comments:*	☐	☐	☐	

                    continued on the following page

continued from the previous page

Procedure 27-1	Able to Perform	Able to Perform with Assistance	Unable to Perform	Initials and Date
24. Grasp top of the probe's stem. *Comments:*	☐	☐	☐	
25. Place tip of thermometer under the client's tongue and along the gumline. *Comments:*	☐	☐	☐	
26. Instruct client to keep mouth closed around thermometer. *Comments:*	☐	☐	☐	
27. Thermometer will signal (beep) when a constant temperature registers. *Comments:*	☐	☐	☐	
28. Read measurement on digital display. Push ejection button to discard disposable sheath and return probe to storage well. *Comments:*	☐	☐	☐	
29. Inform client of temperature reading. *Comments:*	☐	☐	☐	
30. Remove gloves. *Comments:*	☐	☐	☐	
31. Record reading and indicate site. *Comments:*	☐	☐	☐	
32. Return electronic thermometer unit to charging base. *Comments:*	☐	☐	☐	
33. Wash hands. *Comments:*	☐	☐	☐	
Rectal Temperature 34. Repeat steps 1 through 8. *Comments:*	☐	☐	☐	

Procedure 27-1	Able to Perform	Able to Perform with Assistance	Unable to Perform	Initials and Date
35. Place client in the Sims' position with upper knee flexed. Expose only anal area. *Comments:*	☐	☐	☐	
36. Place tissues in easy reach. Apply gloves. *Comments:*	☐	☐	☐	
37. Prepare the thermometer. *Comments:*	☐	☐	☐	
38. Lubricate tip of rectal thermometer or probe with water-soluble lubricant. *Comments:*	☐	☐	☐	
39. Grasp thermometer with one hand and separate buttocks to expose anus with the other. *Comments:*	☐	☐	☐	
40. Instruct client to take a deep breath. Insert thermometer or probe gently into anus. *Comments:*	☐	☐	☐	
41. Hold in place for 2 minutes. *Comments:*	☐	☐	☐	
42. Wipe secretions off glass thermometer with a tissue. Dispose of electronic thermometer cover in waste receptacle. *Comments:*	☐	☐	☐	
43. Read measurement and inform client of temperature reading. *Comments:*	☐	☐	☐	
44. Wipe anal area with tissue to remove lubricant or feces. Cover client. *Comments:*	☐	☐	☐	
45. Cleanse thermometer. *Comments:*	☐	☐	☐	

     continued on the following page

continued from the previous page

Procedure 27-1	Able to Perform	Able to Perform with Assistance	Unable to Perform	Initials and Date
46. Remove and dispose of gloves in appropriate receptacle. Wash hands. *Comments:*	☐	☐	☐	
47. Record reading and indicate site. *Comments:*	☐	☐	☐	
Axillary Temperature 48. Repeat steps 1 through 8. *Comments:*	☐	☐	☐	
49. Remove client's arm and shoulder from sleeve of gown. Avoid exposing chest. *Comments:*	☐	☐	☐	
50. Make sure axillary skin is dry; if necessary, pat dry. *Comments:*	☐	☐	☐	
51. Prepare thermometer. *Comments:*	☐	☐	☐	
52. Place thermometer or probe into center of axilla. Fold client's arm across chest. *Comments:*	☐	☐	☐	
53. Leave glass thermometer in place 6 to 8 minutes. Leave an electronic thermometer in place until signal is heard. *Comments:*	☐	☐	☐	
54. Remove and read thermometer. *Comments:*	☐	☐	☐	
55. Inform client of temperature reading. *Comments:*	☐	☐	☐	
56. Shake glass thermometer down, cleanse, rinse, and return to storage. Dispose of probe cover for electronic thermometer in waste receptacle. *Comments:*	☐	☐	☐	

Procedure 27-1	Able to Perform	Able to Perform with Assistance	Unable to Perform	Initials and Date
57. Assist client with replacing gown. *Comments:*	☐	☐	☐	
58. Record reading and indicate site. *Comments:*	☐	☐	☐	
59. Wash hands. *Comments:*	☐	☐	☐	
Disposable (Chemical Strip) Thermometer 60. Repeat steps 1 through 8. *Comments:*	☐	☐	☐	
61. Apply tape to appropriate skin area, usually forehead. *Comments:*	☐	☐	☐	
62. Observe tape for color changes. *Comments:*	☐	☐	☐	
63. Record reading and indicate method. *Comments:*	☐	☐	☐	
64. Wash hands. *Comments:*	☐	☐	☐	
Tympanic Temperature: Infrared Thermometer 65. Repeat steps 1 through 8. *Comments:*	☐	☐	☐	
66. Position client in Sims' position. *Comments:*	☐	☐	☐	
67. Attach probe cover to tympanic thermometer unit. *Comments:*	☐	☐	☐	
68. Turn client's head to one side. Gently insert probe with firm pressure into ear canal. *Comments:*	☐	☐	☐	

continued on the following page

continued from the previous page

Procedure 27-1	Able to Perform	Able to Perform with Assistance	Unable to Perform	Initials and Date
69. Remove probe after the reading is displayed on digital unit. *Comments:*	☐	☐	☐	
70. Dispose of probe cover appropriately. *Comments:*	☐	☐	☐	
71. Return tympanic thermometer to storage unit. *Comments:*	☐	☐	☐	
72. Record reading and indicate site. *Comments:*	☐	☐	☐	
73. Wash hands. *Comments:*	☐	☐	☐	

_____   _____

Faculty Signature   Date

Checklist for Procedure 27-2   Taking a Pulse

Name _____   Date _____

School _____

Instructor _____

Course _____

Procedure 27-2 Taking a Pulse	Able to Perform	Able to Perform with Assistance	Unable to Perform	Initials and Date
Assessment				
1. Assess client for need to monitor pulse. *Comments:*	☐	☐	☐	
2. Assess for signs of cardiovascular alterations. *Comments:*	☐	☐	☐	
3. Assess for factors that may affect the character of the pulse. *Comments:*	☐	☐	☐	
4. Assess for appropriate site for obtaining pulse. *Comments:*	☐	☐	☐	
5. Assess baseline heart rate and rhythm in the client's chart. *Comments:*	☐	☐	☐	
Planning/Expected Outcomes				
1. Pulse parameters will be within normal range. *Comments:*	☐	☐	☐	
2. The client will be comfortable with the procedure. *Comments:*	☐	☐	☐	
Implementation				
Taking a Radial (Wrist) Pulse 1. Wash hands. *Comments:*	☐	☐	☐	
2. Inform client of the site(s) at which you will measure pulse. *Comments:*	☐	☐	☐	

            continued on the following page

continued from the previous page

Procedure 27-2	Able to Perform	Able to Perform with Assistance	Unable to Perform	Initials and Date
3. Flex client's elbow and place lower part of arm across chest. *Comments:*	☐	☐	☐	
4. Support client's wrist by grasping outer aspect with thumb. *Comments:*	☐	☐	☐	
5. Place your index and middle finger over the radial artery and palpate pulse. *Comments:*	☐	☐	☐	
6. Identify pulse rhythm. *Comments:*	☐	☐	☐	
7. Determine pulse volume. *Comments:*	☐	☐	☐	
8. Count pulse rate by using second hand on a watch. *Comments:*	☐	☐	☐	
Taking an Apical Pulse 9. Wash hands. *Comments:*	☐	☐	☐	
10. Raise client's gown to expose sternum and left side of chest. *Comments:*	☐	☐	☐	
11. Cleanse stethoscope with an alcohol swab. *Comments:*	☐	☐	☐	
12. Put stethoscope around your neck. *Comments:*	☐	☐	☐	
13. Locate apex of heart. *Comments:*	☐	☐	☐	

Procedure 27-2	Able to Perform	Able to Perform with Assistance	Unable to Perform	Initials and Date
14. Instruct client to remain silent so you can listen to his heart. *Comments:*	☐	☐	☐	
15. Put earpieces in your ears and warm stethoscope diaphragm in your hand. *Comments:*	☐	☐	☐	
16. Place diaphragm over the PMI and auscultate for sounds. *Comments:*	☐	☐	☐	
17. Note regularity of rhythm. *Comments:*	☐	☐	☐	
18. Start to count while looking at second hand of watch. Count apical heart rate in all clients for 1 *full* minute. *Comments:*	☐	☐	☐	
19. Share your findings with client. *Comments:*	☐	☐	☐	
20. Record site, rate, rhythm, and number of irregular beats. *Comments:*	☐	☐	☐	
21. Wash hands. *Comments:*	☐	☐	☐	

_____   _____
Faculty Signature   Date

Checklist for Procedure 27-3   Counting Respirations

Name _____   Date _____

School _____

Instructor _____

Course _____

Procedure 27-3 Counting Respirations	Able to Perform	Able to Perform with Assistance	Unable to Perform	Initials and Date
Assessment				
1. Assess the client's chest wall movement. *Comments:*	☐	☐	☐	
2. Assess the rate of respirations. *Comments:*	☐	☐	☐	
3. Assess the depth of the client's breaths. *Comments:*	☐	☐	☐	
4. Assess for risk factors. *Comments:*	☐	☐	☐	
5. Assess for factors that normally influence respirations. *Comments:*	☐	☐	☐	
Planning/Expected Outcomes				
1. An accurate evaluation of the respiratory effort will be obtained. *Comments:*	☐	☐	☐	
2. The respiratory rate and character will be normal. *Comments:*	☐	☐	☐	
Implementation				
1. Wash hands. *Comments:*	☐	☐	☐	
2. Ensure chest movement is visible. *Comments:*	☐	☐	☐	

    continued on the following page

continued from the previous page

Procedure 27-3	Able to Perform	Able to Perform with Assistance	Unable to Perform	Initials and Date
3. Observe one complete respiratory cycle. *Comments:*	☐	☐	☐	
4. Start counting with first inspiration while looking at the second hand of watch. *Comments:*	☐	☐	☐	
5. Observe character of respirations. *Comments:*	☐	☐	☐	
6. Replace client's gown if needed. *Comments:*	☐	☐	☐	
7. Record rate and character of respirations. *Comments:*	☐	☐	☐	
8. Wash hands. *Comments:*	☐	☐	☐	

_____   _____
Faculty Signature   Date

Checklist for Procedure 27-4   Administering Pulse Oximetry

Name _____   Date _____

School _____

Instructor _____

Course _____

Procedure 27-4 Administering Pulse Oximetry	Able to Perform	Able to Perform with Assistance	Unable to Perform	Initials and Date
Assessment				
1. Assess the client's hemoglobin level. *Comments:*	☐	☐	☐	
2. Assess the client's color. *Comments:*	☐	☐	☐	
3. Assess the client's mental status. *Comments:*	☐	☐	☐	
4. Assess the client's pulse rate. *Comments:*	☐	☐	☐	
5. Assess the area where the sensors will be placed. *Comments:*	☐	☐	☐	
Planning/Expected Outcomes				
1. The SaO_2 will be in a normal range for the client. *Comments:*	☐	☐	☐	
2. The client will be alert and oriented. *Comments:*	☐	☐	☐	
3. The client's color will remain normal. *Comments:*	☐	☐	☐	
4. The client will tolerate the placement of sensors. *Comments:*	☐	☐	☐	
5. There will not be any skin irritation at area of sensors. *Comments:*	☐	☐	☐	

                    continued on the following page

continued from the previous page

Procedure 27-4	Able to Perform	Able to Perform with Assistance	Unable to Perform	Initials and Date
Implementation				
1. Wash hands. *Comments:*	☐	☐	☐	
2. Select an appropriate sensor. *Comments:*	☐	☐	☐	
3. Select an appropriate site for the sensor. *Comments:*	☐	☐	☐	
4. Clean the site with an alcohol wipe or soap and water. *Comments:*	☐	☐	☐	
5. Apply the sensor. *Comments:*	☐	☐	☐	
6. Connect the sensor to the oximeter with a sensor cable. Turn on the machine. *Comments:*	☐	☐	☐	
7. Adjust the alarm limits. Adjust volume. *Comments:*	☐	☐	☐	
8. If taking a single reading, note the results. For constant monitoring, move spring sensors every 2 hours and adhesive sensors every 4 hours. *Comments:*	☐	☐	☐	
9. Cover the sensor with a sheet or towel. *Comments:*	☐	☐	☐	
10. Notify the qualified practitioner of abnormal results. *Comments:*	☐	☐	☐	
11. Record the results of O_2 saturation measurements. *Comments:*	☐	☐	☐	

Faculty Signature   Date

Checklist for Procedure 27-5 Taking Blood Pressure

Name _____ Date _____

School _____

Instructor _____

Course _____

Procedure 27-5 Taking Blood Pressure	Able to Perform	Able to Perform with Assistance	Unable to Perform	Initials and Date
Assessment				
1. Assess the condition of the potential blood pressure (BP) site. *Comments:*	☐	☐	☐	
2. Assess the artery for any compromise. *Comments:*	☐	☐	☐	
3. Assess the distal pulse. *Comments:*	☐	☐	☐	
4. Assess the circumference of the extremity. *Comments:*	☐	☐	☐	
5. Assess for factors that affect blood pressure. *Comments:*	☐	☐	☐	
6. Determine client's baseline blood pressure. *Comments:*	☐	☐	☐	
Planning/Expected Outcomes				
1. An accurate estimate of the arterial pressure at diastole and systole will be obtained. *Comments:*	☐	☐	☐	
2. BP is within normal range for the client. *Comments:*	☐	☐	☐	
3. Client will be able to explain why the BP is taken and what it means. *Comments:*	☐	☐	☐	

continued on the following page

continued from the previous page

Procedure 27-5	Able to Perform	Able to Perform with Assistance	Unable to Perform	Initials and Date
Implementation				
Auscultation Method Using Brachial Artery				
1. Wash hands. *Comments:*	☐	☐	☐	
2. Determine which extremity is most appropriate for reading. *Comments:*	☐	☐	☐	
3. Select a cuff size that completely encircles client's upper arm without overlapping bladder ends. *Comments:*	☐	☐	☐	
4. Move client's clothing away from upper aspect of arm. *Comments:*	☐	☐	☐	
5. Position client's arm at heart level, extending elbow with palm turned upward. Have client relax arm and not overly tighten elbow. *Comments:*	☐	☐	☐	
6. Make sure bladder cuff is fully deflated and pump valve moves freely. *Comments:*	☐	☐	☐	
7. Locate brachial artery in the antecubital space. *Comments:*	☐	☐	☐	
8. Apply cuff snugly and smoothly over upper arm. *Comments:*	☐	☐	☐	
9. If using a portable, mercury-filled manometer, position vertically at eye level. *Comments:*	☐	☐	☐	
10. Palpate brachial artery, close valve, and compress bulb to inflate cuff. Slowly release valve, noting reading when pulse is felt again. *Comments:*	☐	☐	☐	

Procedure 27-5	Able to Perform	Able to Perform with Assistance	Unable to Perform	Initials and Date
11. Insert earpieces of stethoscope into ears with a forward tilt. *Comments:*	☐	☐	☐	
12. Relocate brachial pulse and place bell or diaphragm directly over pulse. *Comments:*	☐	☐	☐	
13. Turn valve to close. Inflate cuff to 30 mm Hg above previously noted diminished pulse point. *Comments:*	☐	☐	☐	
14. Slowly open valve so mercury falls 2–3 mm Hg per second. Note manometer readings when sounds appear and disappear. *Comments:*	☐	☐	☐	
15. After the final sound has disappeared, deflate cuff rapidly and completely. *Comments:*	☐	☐	☐	
16. Remove cuff or wait 2 minutes before taking a second reading. *Comments:*	☐	☐	☐	
17. Inform client of reading. *Comments:*	☐	☐	☐	
18. Record reading. *Comments:*	☐	☐	☐	
19. If appropriate, lower bed, raise side rails, and place call light in easy reach. *Comments:*	☐	☐	☐	
20. Put all equipment in proper place. *Comments:*	☐	☐	☐	
21. Wash hands. *Comments:*	☐	☐	☐	

 continued on the following page

continued from the previous page

Procedure 27-5	Able to Perform	Able to Perform with Assistance	Unable to Perform	Initials and Date
Palpation Method Using Brachial or Radial Artery 22. Palpate brachial or radial artery with fingertips. Inflate cuff 30 mm Hg above point at which pulse disappears. *Comments:*	☐	☐	☐	
23. Deflate cuff slowly as you note on the manometer when the pulse is again palpable. *Comments:*	☐	☐	☐	
24. Deflate cuff rapidly and completely. *Comments:*	☐	☐	☐	
25. Remove cuff or wait 2 minutes before taking a second reading. *Comments:*	☐	☐	☐	
26. Inform client of reading. *Comments:*	☐	☐	☐	
27. Record reading. *Comments:*	☐	☐	☐	
28. Wash hands. *Comments:*	☐	☐	☐	

Faculty Signature

Date

Checklist for Procedure 29-1   Performing Venipuncture (Blood Drawing)

Name _____ Date _____

School _____

Instructor _____

Course _____

Procedure 29-1 **Performing Venipuncture (Blood Drawing)**	Able to Perform	Able to Perform with Assistance	Unable to Perform	Initials and Date
Assessment				
1. Determine which test(s) is (are) ordered and any special conditions for the collection or handling of the specimen. *Comments:*	☐	☐	☐	
2. Assess the integrity of the veins to be used in the procedure. *Comments:*	☐	☐	☐	
3. Review the client's medical history. *Comments:*	☐	☐	☐	
4. Determine the client's ability to cooperate with the procedure. *Comments:*	☐	☐	☐	
5. Review the physician's or qualified practitioner's order. *Comments:*	☐	☐	☐	
Planning/Expected Outcomes				
1. Puncture site will not continue to bleed or bruise. *Comments:*	☐	☐	☐	
2. Puncture site will show no evidence of infection. *Comments:*	☐	☐	☐	
3. The specimen will be properly acquired and appropriately handled. *Comments:*	☐	☐	☐	
4. The client will understand the test's purpose and the procedure. *Comments:*	☐	☐	☐	
5. The client will report minimal anxiety from the procedure. *Comments:*	☐	☐	☐	

                    continued on the following page

continued from the previous page

Procedure 29-1	Able to Perform	Able to Perform with Assistance	Unable to Perform	Initials and Date
Implementation				
1. Greet client by name and validate client's identification. *Comments:*	☐	☐	☐	
2. Explain the procedure to the client. *Comments:*	☐	☐	☐	
3. Wash hands. *Comments:*	☐	☐	☐	
4. Close curtain or door. *Comments:*	☐	☐	☐	
5. Bring equipment to bedside or client exam room. *Comments:*	☐	☐	☐	
6. Raise or lower bed/table to a comfortable working height. *Comments:*	☐	☐	☐	
7. Position client's arm. *Comments:*	☐	☐	☐	
8. Apply disposable gloves. *Comments:*	☐	☐	☐	
9. Apply the tourniquet 3 to 4 inches above the venipuncture site. *Comments:*	☐	☐	☐	
10. Check for the distal pulse. *Comments:*	☐	☐	☐	
11. Have client open and close fist several times, leaving fist clenched prior to venipuncture. *Comments:*	☐	☐	☐	
12. Maintain tourniquet only for 1 to 2 minutes. *Comments:*	☐	☐	☐	
13. Identify the best venipuncture site through palpation. *Comments:*	☐	☐	☐	

Procedure 29-1	Able to Perform	Able to Perform with Assistance	Unable to Perform	Initials and Date
14. Select the vein for venipuncture. *Comments:*	☐	☐	☐	

15. Prepare to obtain the blood sample.
  • Syringe method: Have appropriate-sized syringe and needle.
  • Vacutainer method: Attach double-ended needle to Vacutainer holder with the blood specimen tube resting inside the holder, without puncturing the stopper.
Comments:
	☐	☐	☐	

16. Cleanse the site with alcohol swab using a circular motion. *Comments:*	☐	☐	☐	
17. Remove the needle cover and warn the client about the needle stick. *Comments:*	☐	☐	☐	
18. Pull the skin taut below the site. *Comments:*	☐	☐	☐	
19. Hold the needle at 15–30° angle to the skin with the bevel up. *Comments:*	☐	☐	☐	
20. Slowly insert needle. *Comments:*	☐	☐	☐	

21. Technique varies depending on equipment used.
  • Syringe method: Gently pull back on syringe plunger and look for blood return. Obtain desired amount of blood.
  • Vacutainer method: Advance specimen tube onto double-ended needle. After the tube is full of blood, grasp the holder firmly, remove the tube, and insert additional tubes as indicated.
Comments:
	☐	☐	☐	

22. After the specimen is collected, release the tourniquet. *Comments:*	☐	☐	☐	
23. Place gauze over the puncture site, without pressure, and withdraw the needle from the vein. *Comments:*	☐	☐	☐	

                    continued on the following page

continued from the previous page

Procedure 29-1	Able to Perform	Able to Perform with Assistance	Unable to Perform	Initials and Date
24. Apply pressure over the venipuncture site until the bleeding has stopped. Tape the gauze or a Band-Aid over the site. *Comments:*	☐	☐	☐	
25. Syringe method. • Insert the syringe needle into the appropriate collection tubes and allow to fill. *Comments:*	☐	☐	☐	
26. Gently rotate tubes with additives 8–10 times. *Comments:*	☐	☐	☐	
27. Inspect the puncture site for bleeding. Reapply gauze and tape as needed. *Comments:*	☐	☐	☐	
28. Assist client for comfort. Return bed to safe, comfortable position. *Comments:*	☐	☐	☐	
29. Check tubes for external blood and decontaminate as appropriate. *Comments:*	☐	☐	☐	
30. Check for proper labeling and packaging for transport to laboratory. *Comments:*	☐	☐	☐	
31. Dispose of soiled equipment appropriately. *Comments:*	☐	☐	☐	
32. Remove and dispose of gloves. *Comments:*	☐	☐	☐	
33. Wash hands after the procedure. *Comments:*	☐	☐	☐	
34. Send specimens to the laboratory. *Comments:*	☐	☐	☐	

Faculty Signature   Date

Checklist for Procedure 29-2 Skin Puncture

Name _____ Date _____

School _____

Instructor _____

Course _____

Procedure 29-2 Skin Puncture	Able to Perform	Able to Perform with Assistance	Unable to Perform	Initials and Date
Assessment				
1. Assess the condition of the client's skin at the potential puncture site. *Comments:*	☐	☐	☐	
2. Assess the circulation at the potential puncture site. *Comments:*	☐	☐	☐	
3. Assess the client's comfort level regarding the procedure. *Comments:*	☐	☐	☐	
4. Assess the cleanliness of the client's skin. *Comments:*	☐	☐	☐	
Planning/Expected Outcomes				
1. An adequate blood specimen will be obtained. *Comments:*	☐	☐	☐	
2. The client will suffer minimal trauma during specimen collection. *Comments:*	☐	☐	☐	
3. The specimen will be collected and stored in a manner compatible with the ordered tests. *Comments:*	☐	☐	☐	
Implementation				
1. Wash hands. *Comments:*	☐	☐	☐	
2. Check client's identification band, if appropriate. *Comments:*	☐	☐	☐	

  continued on the following page

continued from the previous page

Procedure 29-2	Able to Perform	Able to Perform with Assistance	Unable to Perform	Initials and Date
3. Explain procedure to client. *Comments:*	☐	☐	☐	
4. Prepare supplies, open packages, and label specimen tubes. *Comments:*	☐	☐	☐	
5. Apply gloves. *Comments:*	☐	☐	☐	
6. Select site. *Comments:*	☐	☐	☐	
7. Place the hand or heel in a dependent position. *Comments:*	☐	☐	☐	
8. Place hand towel or absorbent pad under the extremity. *Comments:*	☐	☐	☐	
9. Cleanse puncture site with an antiseptic and allow to dry. *Comments:*	☐	☐	☐	
10. Apply light, kneading pressure above or around the puncture site. *Comments:*	☐	☐	☐	
11. With the sterile lancet at a 90° angle to the skin, use a quick stab to puncture the skin. *Comments:*	☐	☐	☐	
12. Wipe off the first drop of blood with sterile gauze; allow the blood to flow freely. *Comments:*	☐	☐	☐	
13. If blood does not flow freely, gently "milk" the finger or heel from proximal to distal to move blood to the puncture site. (Do not squeeze the finger or heel to obtain a specimen.) *Comments:*	☐	☐	☐	

Procedure 29-2	Able to Perform	Able to Perform with Assistance	Unable to Perform	Initials and Date
14. Collect the blood into the appropriate tube(s). *Comments:*	☐	☐	☐	
15. Apply pressure to the puncture site with sterile gauze. *Comments:*	☐	☐	☐	
16. Place contaminated articles into a sharps container. *Comments:*	☐	☐	☐	
17. Remove and dispose of gloves. Wash hands. *Comments:*	☐	☐	☐	
18. Position client for comfort with call light in reach. *Comments:*	☐	☐	☐	
19. Wash hands. *Comments:*	☐	☐	☐	

_____

Faculty Signature

_____

Date

Checklist for Procedure 29-3   Obtaining a Residual Urine Specimen from an Indwelling Catheter

Name _____ Date _____

School _____

Instructor _____

Course _____

Procedure 29-3 Obtaining a Residual Urine Specimen from an Indwelling Catheter	Able to Perform	Able to Perform with Assistance	Unable to Perform	Initials and Date
Assessment				
1. Identify the purpose of the urine test. *Comments:*	☐	☐	☐	
2. Assess the client's ability to understand purpose of the test. *Comments:*	☐	☐	☐	
3. Identify the type of collecting tubing attached to the indwelling catheter. *Comments:*	☐	☐	☐	
Planning/Expected Outcomes				
1. Client will understand the reason for the specimen. *Comments:*	☐	☐	☐	
2. Specimen will be obtained in the proper container in a timely manner. *Comments:*	☐	☐	☐	
3. Specimen will remain uncontaminated. *Comments:*	☐	☐	☐	
Implementation				
1. Wash hands. *Comments:*	☐	☐	☐	
2. Check physician's or qualified practitioner's order. *Comments:*	☐	☐	☐	
3. Explain procedure to the client and provide privacy. *Comments:*	☐	☐	☐	

continued on the following page

continued from the previous page

Procedure 29-3	Able to Perform	Able to Perform with Assistance	Unable to Perform	Initials and Date
4. Check for urine in the tubing. *Comments:*	☐	☐	☐	
5. If more urine is needed, clamp the tubing for 10 to 15 minutes. *Comments:*	☐	☐	☐	
6. Put on clean gloves. *Comments:*	☐	☐	☐	
7. Clean sample port or the catheter with a Betadine swab. *Comments:*	☐	☐	☐	
8. Insert sterile needle and syringe into the sample port or catheter at a 45° angle and withdraw 10 ml of urine. *Comments:*	☐	☐	☐	
9. Put urine into sterile container and close tightly. *Comments:*	☐	☐	☐	
10. Remove clamp and rearrange tubing, avoiding dependent loops. *Comments:*	☐	☐	☐	
11. Label specimen container, put it in a plastic bag, and send to the laboratory. *Comments:*	☐	☐	☐	
12. Wash hands *Comments:*	☐	☐	☐	
13. Record procedure on flow sheet or approved agency form. *Comments:*	☐	☐	☐	

Faculty Signature   Date

Checklist for Procedure 30-1 Administering Oral, Sublingual, and Buccal Medications

Name _____ Date _____

School _____

Instructor _____

Course _____

Procedure 30-1 Administering Oral, Sublingual, and Buccal Medications	Able to Perform	Able to Perform with Assistance	Unable to Perform	Initials and Date
Assessment				
1. Review each drug to be given. *Comments:*	☐	☐	☐	
2. Assess the client's condition and the written order. *Comments:*	☐	☐	☐	
3. Assess the client's ability to swallow food and fluid. *Comments:*	☐	☐	☐	
4. Assess for any contraindications for oral medication. *Comments:*	☐	☐	☐	
5. Assess the client's medical record for allergies. *Comments:*	☐	☐	☐	
6. Assess the client's knowledge about the use of medications. *Comments:*	☐	☐	☐	
7. Assess the client's age. *Comments:*	☐	☐	☐	
8. Assess the client's need for fluids. *Comments:*	☐	☐	☐	
9. Assess the client's ability to sit or turn to the side. *Comments:*	☐	☐	☐	
Planning/Expected Outcomes				
1. The client will swallow the prescribed medication. *Comments:*	☐	☐	☐	

 continued on the following page

continued from the previous page

Procedure 30-1	Able to Perform	Able to Perform with Assistance	Unable to Perform	Initials and Date
2. The client will understand the medication's purpose and schedule. *Comments:*	☐	☐	☐	
3. The client will have no discomfort or alterations in function. *Comments:*	☐	☐	☐	
4. The client will show the desired response to the medication. *Comments:*	☐	☐	☐	
Implementation				
1. Wash hands and put on clean gloves. *Comments:*	☐	☐	☐	
2. Arrange the medication tray and cups. *Comments:*	☐	☐	☐	
3. Unlock the medication cart or log on to the computer. *Comments:*	☐	☐	☐	
4. Prepare medication for one client at a time using the five rights. *Comments:*	☐	☐	☐	
5. To prepare a tablet or capsule: • Pour into the medication cup without touching it. • Scored tablets may be broken or crushed. • Do not open unit-dose tablets. *Comments:*	☐	☐	☐	
6. To prepare a liquid medication: • Remove the bottle cap and place cap upside down. • Pour medication at eye level to the desired dose. *Comments:*	☐	☐	☐	
7. To prepare a narcotic, obtain the key and sign out the dose. *Comments:*	☐	☐	☐	

Procedure 30-1	Able to Perform	Able to Perform with Assistance	Unable to Perform	Initials and Date
8. Check expiration date on all medications. • Double-check the medication administration record (MAR) with the prepared drugs and place with the client's medications. • Return stock medications to their shelf or drawer. *Comments:*	☐	☐	☐	
9. Administer medications to client. • Observe the correct time to give the medication. • Identify the client. • Check to ensure that this is the correct medication type and dosage. • Assess suitability of the form of the medication. • Perform any assessment required for specific medications. • Explain the purpose of the drug and answer any questions. • Assist the client to a sitting or lateral position. • Allow client to hold the tablet or medication cup. • Give a glass of liquid, and straw if needed. • For *sublingual* medications, instruct client to dissolve medication under the tongue. • For *buccal* medications, instruct the client to dissolve medication in the mouth against the cheek. • For medications given through a *nasogastric tube,* crush tablets or open capsules and dissolve with warm water. • Remain with the client until each medication has been swallowed or dissolved. • Assist the client into a comfortable position. *Comments:*	☐	☐	☐	
10. Dispose of soiled supplies and wash hands. *Comments:*	☐	☐	☐	
11. Record the time and route on the MAR. *Comments:*	☐	☐	☐	
12. Return the cart; clean and restock as needed. *Comments:*	☐	☐	☐	

Faculty Signature   Date

Checklist for Procedure 30-2　Withdrawing Medication from an Ampoule

Name _____ Date _____

School _____

Instructor _____

Course _____

Procedure 30-2 Withdrawing Medication from an Ampoule	Able to Perform	Able to Perform with Assistance	Unable to Perform	Initials and Date
Assessment				
1. Identify the correct ampoule. *Comments:*	☐	☐	☐	
2. Assess the syringe, filter needle, and injection needle. *Comments:*	☐	☐	☐	
3. Assess the fluid in the ampoule. *Comments:*	☐	☐	☐	
4. Identify the medication's intended action, purpose, and nursing implications. *Comments:*	☐	☐	☐	
Planning/Expected Outcomes				
1. The correct medication ampoule will be selected. *Comments:*	☐	☐	☐	
2. The medication will be drawn into an appropriate syringe. *Comments:*	☐	☐	☐	
3. Microorganisms will not be introduced into the sterile system. *Comments:*	☐	☐	☐	
4. Foreign objects will not be introduced into the sterile system. *Comments:*	☐	☐	☐	
Implementation				
1. Wash hands. *Comments:*	☐	☐	☐	

　　　　continued on the following page

continued from the previous page

Procedure 30-2	Able to Perform	Able to Perform with Assistance	Unable to Perform	Initials and Date
2. Select appropriate ampoule. *Comments:*	☐	☐	☐	
3. Select syringe with filter needle. *Comments:*	☐	☐	☐	
4. Obtain a sterile gauze pad. *Comments:*	☐	☐	☐	
5. Select and set aside the appropriate length of needle for planned injection. *Comments:*	☐	☐	☐	
6. Clear a work space. *Comments:*	☐	☐	☐	
7. Observe ampoule for location of the fluid. *Comments:*	☐	☐	☐	
8. If fluid is trapped in the top, flick the neck of the ampoule. *Comments:*	☐	☐	☐	
9. Wrap the sterile gauze pad around the neck and snap off the top in an outward motion. *Comments:*	☐	☐	☐	
10. Invert ampoule, place the needle into the liquid, and withdraw fluid into the syringe. *Comments:*	☐	☐	☐	
11. Alternately, place the ampoule on the counter, hold and tilt slightly. Insert the needle into liquid and draw liquid into the syringe. *Comments:*	☐	☐	☐	
12. Remove the filter needle and replace with the injection needle. *Comments:*	☐	☐	☐	

Procedure 30-2	Able to Perform	Able to Perform with Assistance	Unable to Perform	Initials and Date
13. Dispose of filter needle and glass ampoule appropriately. *Comments:*	☐	☐	☐	
14. Label the syringe with drug, dose, date, and time. For a single-dose vial, discard unused portion of medication as directed by agency policy. *Comments:*	☐	☐	☐	
15. Wash hands. *Comments:*	☐	☐	☐	

Faculty Signature

Date

Checklist for Procedure 30-3   Withdrawing Medication from a Vial

Name _____   Date _____

School _____

Instructor _____

Course _____

Procedure 30-3 Withdrawing Medication from a Vial	Able to Perform	Able to Perform with Assistance	Unable to Perform	Initials and Date
Assessment				
1. Assess the expiration date on the vial to be sure it is current. *Comments:*	☐	☐	☐	
2. Assess the contents of the vial for the correct medication and dosage. *Comments:*	☐	☐	☐	
3. Assess the contents of the vial for color, consistency, and debris. *Comments:*	☐	☐	☐	
4. Assess the integrity of the vial and the stopper. *Comments:*	☐	☐	☐	
5. Assess the integrity of the syringe and needle that will be used. *Comments:*	☐	☐	☐	
Planning/Expected Outcomes				
1. The correct medication will be drawn from the vial using sterile technique. *Comments:*	☐	☐	☐	
2. The correct dose will be drawn from the vial. *Comments:*	☐	☐	☐	
3. The remaining contents of multiuse vials will not be contaminated. *Comments:*	☐	☐	☐	
4. The date the vial was opened will be marked on the vial in ink. *Comments:*	☐	☐	☐	

                      continued on the following page

continued from the previous page

Procedure 30-3	Able to Perform	Able to Perform with Assistance	Unable to Perform	Initials and Date
Implementation				
1. Wash hands. Apply gloves if desired. *Comments:*	☐	☐	☐	
2. Select the appropriate vial. *Comments:*	☐	☐	☐	
3. Verify physician's or qualified practitioner's orders. *Comments:*	☐	☐	☐	
4. Check expiration date. *Comments:*	☐	☐	☐	
5. Determine the medication route and select the appropriate size syringe and needle. *Comments:*	☐	☐	☐	
6. Withdraw the plunger to the desired volume of medication. *Comments:*	☐	☐	☐	
7. Clean the rubber top of the vial with an alcohol pad. *Comments:*	☐	☐	☐	
8. Remove the cap from the needle. *Comments:*	☐	☐	☐	
9. Lay the needle cap on a clean surface. *Comments:*	☐	☐	☐	
10. Placing the needle in the center of the vial, inject air slowly. *Comments:*	☐	☐	☐	
11. Invert the vial and withdraw the medication. *Comments:*	☐	☐	☐	
12. Determine that the appropriate dose/volume has been reached. *Comments:*	☐	☐	☐	

Procedure 30-3	Able to Perform	Able to Perform with Assistance	Unable to Perform	Initials and Date
13. Slowly withdraw the needle from the vial. *Comments:*	☐	☐	☐	
14. Using ink, mark the current date, time, and initials on the vial. For a single-dose vial, discard unused portion of medication as directed by agency policy. *Comments:*	☐	☐	☐	
15. Label the syringe with drug, dose, date, and time. *Comments:*	☐	☐	☐	
16. Wash hands. *Comments:*	☐	☐	☐	

Faculty Signature

Date

Checklist for Procedure 30-4   Mixing Medications from Two Vials into One Syringe

Name _____ Date _____

School _____

Instructor _____

Course _____

Procedure 30-4 Mixing Medications from Two Vials into One Syringe	Able to Perform	Able to Perform with Assistance	Unable to Perform	Initials and Date
Assessment				
1. Identify the medications, dosage, and route ordered and the normal dosage and route. *Comments:*	☐	☐	☐	
2. Consider whether the order of drawing up medications makes a difference. *Comments:*	☐	☐	☐	
3. Assess client's knowledge regarding this skill if the client will be doing this at home. *Comments:*	☐	☐	☐	
Planning/Expected Outcomes				
1. The ordered medications will be drawn up using sterile technique. *Comments:*	☐	☐	☐	
2. The correct dose of medication will be drawn from the vials. *Comments:*	☐	☐	☐	
3. The remaining contents of multiuse vials will not be contaminated. *Comments:*	☐	☐	☐	
4. If needed, client will be instructed in performing this skill. *Comments:*	☐	☐	☐	
Implementation				
1. Check MAR against the written orders. *Comments:*	☐	☐	☐	
2. Check for drug allergies. *Comments:*	☐	☐	☐	

                    continued on the following page

continued from the previous page

Procedure 30-4	Able to Perform	Able to Perform with Assistance	Unable to Perform	Initials and Date
3. Wash your hands. *Comments:*	☐	☐	☐	
4. Gather the equipment needed. Prepare the medication for one client at a time. *Comments:*	☐	☐	☐	
5. Check the need for one medication to be drawn up before the other. *Comments:*	☐	☐	☐	
6. Determine the total volume of the combined medications. *Comments:*	☐	☐	☐	
7. Swab the top of each vial with alcohol. *Comments:*	☐	☐	☐	
8. Draw air into the syringe equal to the volume to be drawn up from the second vial. Inject the air into the second vial and remove the syringe and needle from the vial. *Comments:*	☐	☐	☐	
9. Draw air into the syringe equal to the volume to be drawn up from the first vial. Inject air into the first vial. Keep the needle and syringe in the vial. *Comments:*	☐	☐	☐	
10. Withdraw the correct amount of medication from the first vial. *Comments:*	☐	☐	☐	
11. Remove the syringe from the first vial and insert it into the second vial. Withdraw medication from second vial to the volume total of both medications summed together. *Comments:*	☐	☐	☐	
12. Follow the institutional policy regarding recapping needles. *Comments:*	☐	☐	☐	
13. Wash hands. *Comments:*	☐	☐	☐	

_____   _____
Faculty Signature   Date

Checklist for Procedure 30-5   Administering an Intradermal Injection

Name _____ Date _____

School _____

Instructor _____

Course _____

Procedure 30-5 **Administering an Intradermal Injection**	Able to Perform	Able to Perform with Assistance	Unable to Perform	Initials and Date
Assessment				
1. Review physician's or qualified practitioner's order. *Comments:*	☐	☐	☐	
2. Review information regarding the expected outcomes. *Comments:*	☐	☐	☐	
3. Assess for the indications for intradermal injection. *Comments:*	☐	☐	☐	
4. Check the expiration date of the medication vial. *Comments:*	☐	☐	☐	
5. Assess client's knowledge regarding the medication to be received. *Comments:*	☐	☐	☐	
6. Assess the client's response to discussion about an injection. *Comments:*	☐	☐	☐	
Planning/Expected Outcomes				
1. The client will experience minimal pain at the injection site. *Comments:*	☐	☐	☐	
2. The client will experience no allergic reaction or side effects. *Comments:*	☐	☐	☐	
3. The client will be able to explain the significance of a skin reaction. *Comments:*	☐	☐	☐	
4. The client will keep follow-up appointments. *Comments:*	☐	☐	☐	

   continued on the following page

continued from the previous page

Procedure 30-5	Able to Perform	Able to Perform with Assistance	Unable to Perform	Initials and Date
Implementation				
1. Wash hands and put on clean gloves. *Comments:*	☐	☐	☐	
2. Provide privacy. Identify client. *Comments:*	☐	☐	☐	
3. Select injection site. *Comments:*	☐	☐	☐	
4. Select one-quarter- to five-eighths-inch 25- to 27-gauge needle. *Comments:*	☐	☐	☐	
5. Assist client into a comfortable position. • Relax the arm with forearm extended on a flat surface. • Distract client by talking about an interesting subject. *Comments:*	☐	☐	☐	
6. Use antiseptic swab in a circular motion to clean skin at site. *Comments:*	☐	☐	☐	
7. Pull cap from needle. *Comments:*	☐	☐	☐	
8. Administer injection: • Stretch skin over site with forefinger and thumb. • Insert needle slowly until resistance is felt; then advance to no more than an eighth of an inch. • Slowly inject the medication. • Note a small bleb forming under the skin surface. *Comments:*	☐	☐	☐	
9. Withdraw the needle, applying gentle pressure with the swab. *Comments:*	☐	☐	☐	
10. Do not massage the site. *Comments:*	☐	☐	☐	

Procedure 30-5	Able to Perform	Able to Perform with Assistance	Unable to Perform	Initials and Date
11. Assist the client to a comfortable position. *Comments:*	☐	☐	☐	
12. Discard the uncapped needle and syringe safely. *Comments:*	☐	☐	☐	
13. Remove gloves and wash hands. *Comments:*	☐	☐	☐	
14. Document procedure if indicated. *Comments:*	☐	☐	☐	

_____   _____

Faculty Signature   Date

Checklist for Procedure 30-6 Administering a Subcutaneous Injection

Name _____ Date _____

School _____

Instructor _____

Course _____

Procedure 30-6 Administering a Subcutaneous Injection	Able to Perform	Able to Perform with Assistance	Unable to Perform	Initials and Date
Assessment				
1. Review physician's or qualified practitioner's order. *Comments:*	☐	☐	☐	
2. Review information regarding the drug ordered. *Comments:*	☐	☐	☐	
3. Assess client for factors that may influence an injection. *Comments:*	☐	☐	☐	
4. Assess for previous subcutaneous injections. *Comments:*	☐	☐	☐	
5. Assess for the indications for subcutaneous injection. *Comments:*	☐	☐	☐	
6. Assess the client's age. *Comments:*	☐	☐	☐	
7. Assess client's knowledge regarding the medication. *Comments:*	☐	☐	☐	
8. Assess the client's response to discussion about an injection. *Comments:*	☐	☐	☐	
Planning/Expected Outcomes				
1. The client will experience minimal pain or burning at the injection site. *Comments:*	☐	☐	☐	
2. The client will experience no allergic reaction or other side effects. *Comments:*	☐	☐	☐	

 continued on the following page

continued from the previous page

Procedure 30-6	Able to Perform	Able to Perform with Assistance	Unable to Perform	Initials and Date
3. The client will be able to explain the purpose, action, schedule, and side effects of the medication. *Comments:*	☐	☐	☐	

Implementation

	Able to Perform	Able to Perform with Assistance	Unable to Perform	Initials and Date
1. Wash hands and put on clean gloves. *Comments:*	☐	☐	☐	
2. Provide privacy. Identify client. *Comments:*	☐	☐	☐	
3. Select injection site. *Comments:*	☐	☐	☐	
4. Select needle size. *Comments:*	☐	☐	☐	
5. Assist client into a comfortable position. Distract client. *Comments:*	☐	☐	☐	
6. Use antiseptic swab to clean skin at site. *Comments:*	☐	☐	☐	
7. While holding swab between fingers, pull cap from needle. *Comments:*	☐	☐	☐	
8. Administer injection: • Hold syringe like a dart. • Pinch skin with nondominant hand. • Inject needle quickly and firmly. • Release the skin. • Grasp the lower end of the syringe with one hand, and position other hand at the end of the plunger. • Pull back on the plunger. If no blood appears, slowly inject the medication. *Comments:*	☐	☐	☐	
9. Withdraw the needle while applying pressure with the swab. *Comments:*	☐	☐	☐	

Procedure 30-6	Able to Perform	Able to Perform with Assistance	Unable to Perform	Initials and Date
10. Gently massage the site unless massage is contraindicated for prescribed medication. *Comments:*	☐	☐	☐	
11. Assist the client to a comfortable position. *Comments:*	☐	☐	☐	
12. Discard the uncapped needle and syringe appropriately. *Comments:*	☐	☐	☐	
13. Remove gloves and wash hands. *Comments:*	☐	☐	☐	

_____   _____

Faculty Signature   Date

Checklist for Procedure 30-7 Administering an Intramuscular Injection

Name _____ Date _____

School _____

Instructor _____

Course _____

Procedure 30-7 **Administering an Intramuscular Injection**	Able to Perform	Able to Perform with Assistance	Unable to Perform	Initials and Date
Assessment				
1. Review physician's or qualified practitioner's order. *Comments:*	☐	☐	☐	
2. Review information regarding the drug ordered. *Comments:*	☐	☐	☐	
3. Assess client for factors that may influence an injection. *Comments:*	☐	☐	☐	
4. Assess for previous intramuscular injections. *Comments:*	☐	☐	☐	
5. Assess for the indications for intramuscular injections. *Comments:*	☐	☐	☐	
6. Assess the client's age. *Comments:*	☐	☐	☐	
7. Assess client's knowledge regarding the medication to be received. *Comments:*	☐	☐	☐	
8. Assess the client's response to discussion about an injection. *Comments:*	☐	☐	☐	
Planning/Expected Outcomes				
1. The client will experience minimal pain at the injection site. *Comments:*	☐	☐	☐	
2. The client will experience no allergic reaction or other side effects. *Comments:*	☐	☐	☐	

 continued on the following page

continued from the previous page

Procedure 30-7	Able to Perform	Able to Perform with Assistance	Unable to Perform	Initials and Date
3. The client will be able to explain the action, side effects, dosage, and schedule of the medication. *Comments:*	☐	☐	☐	
Implementation				
1. Wash hands and put on clean gloves. *Comments:*	☐	☐	☐	
2. Provide privacy. Identify client. *Comments:*	☐	☐	☐	
3. Select injection site. *Comments:*	☐	☐	☐	
4. Select needle size. *Comments:*	☐	☐	☐	
5. Assist client into a comfortable position. *Comments:*	☐	☐	☐	
6. Use antiseptic swab to clean skin at site. *Comments:*	☐	☐	☐	
7. While holding swab between fingers, pull cap from needle. *Comments:*	☐	☐	☐	
8. Administer injection: • Hold syringe between thumb and forefinger, like a dart. • Spread skin tightly. • Inject needle quickly and firmly. • Release the skin. • Grasp the lower end of the syringe with one hand and position other hand at the end of the plunger. • Pull back on the plunger. If no blood appears, inject the medication. *Comments:*	☐	☐	☐	
9. Withdraw the needle while applying pressure with the swab. *Comments:*	☐	☐	☐	

Procedure 30-7	Able to Perform	Able to Perform with Assistance	Unable to Perform	Initials and Date
10. Gently massage the site. *Comments:*	☐	☐	☐	
11. Assist the client to a comfortable position. *Comments:*	☐	☐	☐	
12. Discard the uncapped needle and syringe appropriately. *Comments:*	☐	☐	☐	
13. Remove gloves and wash hands. *Comments:*	☐	☐	☐	

_____   _____

Faculty Signature   Date

Checklist for Procedure 30-8   Administering Medications via Secondary Administration Sets (Piggyback)

Name _____ Date _____

School _____

Instructor _____

Course _____

Procedure 30-8 **Administering Medications via Secondary Administration Sets (Piggyback)**	Able to Perform	Able to Perform with Assistance	Unable to Perform	Initials and Date
Assessment				
1. Check the order for the medication, dosage, time, and route of administration. *Comments:*	☐	☐	☐	
2. Review information regarding the drug. *Comments:*	☐	☐	☐	
3. Determine the additives in the solution of an existing IV line. *Comments:*	☐	☐	☐	
4. Assess the placement of the IV catheter in the vein. *Comments:*	☐	☐	☐	
5. Assess the skin at the IV site. *Comments:*	☐	☐	☐	
6. Check the client's drug allergy history. *Comments:*	☐	☐	☐	
7. Assess the client's understanding of the purpose of the medication. *Comments:*	☐	☐	☐	
8. Assess the compatibility of the piggyback IV medication with the primary IV solution. *Comments:*	☐	☐	☐	
Planning/Expected Outcomes				
1. The drug is infused into the vein without complications. *Comments:*	☐	☐	☐	
2. The IV site remains free of swelling and inflammation. *Comments:*	☐	☐	☐	

continued on the following page

continued from the previous page

Procedure 30-8	Able to Perform	Able to Perform with Assistance	Unable to Perform	Initials and Date
3. The client will be able to discuss the purpose of the drug. *Comments:*	☐	☐	☐	
Implementation				
1. Check physician's or qualified practitioner's order. *Comments:*	☐	☐	☐	
2. Wash hands and put on clean gloves. *Comments:*	☐	☐	☐	
3. Check client's identification bracelet. *Comments:*	☐	☐	☐	
4. Explain procedure and reason drug is being given. *Comments:*	☐	☐	☐	
5. Prepare medication bag. • Close clamp on tubing of secondary infusion set. • Spike medication bag with secondary infusion tubing. • Open clamp. • Allow tubing to fill with solution. *Comments:*	☐	☐	☐	
6. Hang piggyback medication bag above level of primary IV bag. *Comments:*	☐	☐	☐	
7. Connect piggyback tubing to primary tubing at Y-port. • For needleless system, remove port cap and connect tubing. • If a needle is used, clean port with antiseptic swab and insert small-gauge needle into center of port. • Secure tubing with adhesive tape. *Comments:*	☐	☐	☐	
8. Administer the medication. • Check the prescribed length of time for the infusion. • Regulate the flow rate of the piggyback. • Observe that primary infusion has stopped during drug administration. *Comments:*	☐	☐	☐	

Procedure 30-8	Able to Perform	Able to Perform with Assistance	Unable to Perform	Initials and Date
9. Check primary infusion line when medication is finished. 　• Regulate primary infusion rate. 　• Leave secondary bag and tubing in place. *Comments:*	☐	☐	☐	
10. Remove gloves and dispose of contaminated materials appropriately. *Comments:*	☐	☐	☐	
11. Wash hands. *Comments:*	☐	☐	☐	

Faculty Signature　　　　　　　　　　　　　　　　　　Date

Checklist for Procedure 30-9   Administering Ear and Eye Medications

Name _____ Date _____

School _____

Instructor _____

Course _____

Procedure 30-9 **Administering Ear and Eye Medications**	Able to Perform	Able to Perform with Assistance	Unable to Perform	Initials and Date
Assessment				
1. Assess the five rights. *Comments:*	☐	☐	☐	
2. Assess the condition of the client's eyes and/or ears. *Comments:*	☐	☐	☐	
3. Assess the medication order. *Comments:*	☐	☐	☐	
Planning/Expected Outcomes				
1. The client will receive the medication according to the five rights. *Comments:*	☐	☐	☐	
2. The client will encounter the minimum of discomfort. *Comments:*	☐	☐	☐	
3. The client will receive maximum benefit from the medication. *Comments:*	☐	☐	☐	
Implementation				
Eye Medication				
1. Check for allergies or other contraindications. *Comments:*	☐	☐	☐	
2. Gather the necessary equipment. *Comments:*	☐	☐	☐	
3. Follow the five rights of drug administration. *Comments:*	☐	☐	☐	

                    continued on the following page

continued from the previous page

Procedure 30-9	Able to Perform	Able to Perform with Assistance	Unable to Perform	Initials and Date
4. Place the medication on a clean surface in the client's room. *Comments:*	☐	☐	☐	
5. Check client's identification armband. *Comments:*	☐	☐	☐	
6. Explain the procedure; assist the client as needed. *Comments:*	☐	☐	☐	
7. Wash hands. Apply nonsterile gloves if needed. *Comments:*	☐	☐	☐	
8. Place client in a supine position with the head slightly hyperextended. *Comments:*	☐	☐	☐	
Instilling Eyedrops 9. Remove cap from bottle and place cap on its side. *Comments:*	☐	☐	☐	
10. Squeeze the prescribed dose of medication into the eyedropper. *Comments:*	☐	☐	☐	
11. Place a tissue below the lower lid. *Comments:*	☐	☐	☐	
12. Hold eyedropper above the eyeball. *Comments:*	☐	☐	☐	
13. Expose lower conjunctival sac by pulling down on cheek. *Comments:*	☐	☐	☐	
14. While client looks up, drop prescribed dose into center of conjunctival sac. *Comments:*	☐	☐	☐	
15. While client closes and moves eyes, place fingers on either side of the client's nose. *Comments:*	☐	☐	☐	

Procedure 30-9	Able to Perform	Able to Perform with Assistance	Unable to Perform	Initials and Date
16. Remove gloves; wash hands. *Comments:*	☐	☐	☐	
17. Record route, site, and time on the MAR. *Comments:*	☐	☐	☐	
Eye Ointment Application 18. Repeat steps 1 through 8. *Comments:*	☐	☐	☐	
Lower Lid 19. • Separate client's eyelids and grasp lower lid; exert downward pressure over the cheek. • Instruct the client to look up. • Apply eye ointment along inside edge of the lower eyelid from inner to outer canthus. *Comments:*	☐	☐	☐	
Upper Lid 20. • Instruct client to look down. • Grasp lashes near center of upper lid and draw lid up and away from eyeball. • Squeeze ointment along upper lid starting at inner canthus. *Comments:*	☐	☐	☐	
21. Repeat steps 16 and 17. *Comments:*	☐	☐	☐	
Medication Disk 22. Repeat steps 1 through 8. *Comments:*	☐	☐	☐	
23. Open package and press sterile gloved finger against the disk. *Comments:*	☐	☐	☐	
24. Instruct the client to look up. *Comments:*	☐	☐	☐	

continued on the following page

continued from the previous page

Procedure 30-9	Able to Perform	Able to Perform with Assistance	Unable to Perform	Initials and Date
25. Pull the client's lower eyelid down and place the disk horizontally in the conjunctival sac. • Pull the lower eyelid out, up, and over the disk. • Instruct the client to blink several times. • If disk is still visible, repeat steps. • Instruct the client to press the fingers against the closed lids. • If the disk falls out, rinse it under cool water and reinsert. *Comments:*	☐	☐	☐	
26. If the disk is prescribed for both eyes, repeat steps 23 through 25. *Comments:*	☐	☐	☐	
27. Repeat steps 16 and 17. *Comments:*	☐	☐	☐	
Removing an Eye Medication Disk 28. Repeat steps 3 and 5 through 8. *Comments:*	☐	☐	☐	
29. Remove the disk. • Invert the lower eyelid and identify the disk. • If in the upper eye, stroke the client's closed eyelid to move the disk to the corner of eye. • Slide the disk onto the lower eyelid and out of the client's eye. *Comments:*	☐	☐	☐	
30. Remove gloves; wash hands. *Comments:*	☐	☐	☐	
31. Record on the MAR the removal of the disk. *Comments:*	☐	☐	☐	
Ear Medication 1. Check with client and chart for any known allergies. *Comments:*	☐	☐	☐	
2. Check the MAR against the written orders. *Comments:*	☐	☐	☐	

Procedure 30-9	Able to Perform	Able to Perform with Assistance	Unable to Perform	Initials and Date
3. Wash hands. *Comments:*	☐	☐	☐	
4. Calculate the dose. *Comments:*	☐	☐	☐	
5. Use the identification armband to properly identify the client. *Comments:*	☐	☐	☐	
6. Explain the procedure to the client. *Comments:*	☐	☐	☐	
7. Place the client in a side-lying position with the affected ear facing up. *Comments:*	☐	☐	☐	
8. Straighten the ear canal by pulling the pinna. *Comments:*	☐	☐	☐	
9. Instill the drops into the ear canal. *Comments:*	☐	☐	☐	
10. Ask the client to maintain the position for 2 to 3 minutes. *Comments:*	☐	☐	☐	
11. Place a cotton ball on the outermost part of the canal. *Comments:*	☐	☐	☐	
12. Wash hands. *Comments:*	☐	☐	☐	
13. Document the drug, amount, time, and ear medicated. *Comments:*	☐	☐	☐	

Faculty Signature　　　　　　　　　　　　　　　　Date

Checklist for Procedure 30-10   Administering Nasal Medications

Name _____ Date _____

School _____

Instructor _____

Course _____

Procedure 30-10 Administering Nasal Medications	Able to Perform	Able to Perform with Assistance	Unable to Perform	Initials and Date
Assessment				
1. Assess the client's nasal congestion and nasal obstruction. *Comments:*	☐	☐	☐	
2. Assess the client's discharge and nasal mucosa. *Comments:*	☐	☐	☐	
3. Assess the client's pain and/or discomfort level in the sinuses. *Comments:*	☐	☐	☐	
4. Assess the client for adverse systemic conditions. *Comments:*	☐	☐	☐	
Planning/Expected Outcomes				
1. The client will be free of nasal congestion. *Comments:*	☐	☐	☐	
2. The client will be free of nasal discharge and odor. *Comments:*	☐	☐	☐	
3. The client will breathe freely through the nasal passages. *Comments:*	☐	☐	☐	
4. The client will be free of sinus pain and nasal pain. *Comments:*	☐	☐	☐	
5. The client's nasal passages will be moist and pink. *Comments:*	☐	☐	☐	

    continued on the following page

continued from the previous page

Procedure 30-10	Able to Perform	Able to Perform with Assistance	Unable to Perform	Initials and Date
Implementation				
1. Wash hands. Wear a mask if needed. *Comments:*	☐	☐	☐	
2. Explain the purpose of the medication and the desired head position. *Comments:*	☐	☐	☐	
3. Explain the sensation of the medications. *Comments:*	☐	☐	☐	
4. If a nasal inhaler is used, explain how inhalers work. Follow the five rights. *Comments:*	☐	☐	☐	
5. Have the client blow nose and assume desired position. Squeeze nose drops into dropper. *Comments:*	☐	☐	☐	
6. Have the client exhale and close one nostril. *Comments:*	☐	☐	☐	
7. Have client inhale while medication is sprayed into the first nostril. If drops are used, insert dropper and instill the prescribed dosage. *Comments:*	☐	☐	☑	
8. Have client blot excess drainage; do not blow nose. *Comments:*	☐	☐	☐	
9. Repeat the procedure on the other nostril. *Comments:*	☐	☐	☐	
10. Help the client resume a comfortable position. If nose drops are used, have client maintain a therapeutic position. *Comments:*	☐	☐	☐	
11. Dispose of soiled articles appropriately. Wash hands. *Comments:*	☐	☐	☐	

Procedure 30-10	Able to Perform	Able to Perform with Assistance	Unable to Perform	Initials and Date
12. Evaluate the effect of the medication in 15 to 20 minutes. *Comments:*	☐	☐	☐	
13. Wash hands. *Comments:*	☐	☐	☐	

_____   _____

Faculty Signature   Date

Checklist for Procedure 30-11 Teaching Self-Administration with a Metered-Dose Inhaler (MDI)

Name _____ Date _____

School _____

Instructor _____

Course _____

Procedure 30-11 Teaching Self-Administration with a Metered-Dose Inhaler (MDI)	Able to Perform	Able to Perform with Assistance	Unable to Perform	Initials and Date
Assessment				
1. Assess the client's respiratory status. *Comments:*	☐	☐	☐	
2. Evaluate the history of this episode of the client's distress. *Comments:*	☐	☐	☐	
3. Assess the client's ability to use the metered-dose inhaler (MDI). *Comments:*	☐	☐	☐	
4. Assess the medication(s) currently ordered. *Comments:*	☐	☐	☐	
5. Assess the medications the client is currently taking. *Comments:*	☐	☐	☐	
6. Assess the client's knowledge of the medications and the delivery method. *Comments:*	☐	☐	☐	
Planning/Expected Outcomes				
1. The client will experience improved gas exchange. *Comments:*	☐	☐	☐	
2. The client's breathing pattern will become effective. *Comments:*	☐	☐	☐	
3. The client will understand the need for the medication and the delivery system. *Comments:*	☐	☐	☐	

continued on the following page

continued from the previous page

Procedure 30-11	Able to Perform	Able to Perform with Assistance	Unable to Perform	Initials and Date
4. The client will not experience any adverse effects. *Comments:*	☐	☐	☐	
5. The client's anxiety level will decrease following treatment. *Comments:*	☐	☐	☐	

Implementation

Metered-Dose Inhaler

	Able to Perform	Able to Perform with Assistance	Unable to Perform	Initials and Date
1. Check for drug allergies and hypersensitivity. *Comments:*	☐	☐	☐	
2. Check the MAR against the orders. *Comments:*	☐	☐	☐	
3. Wash hands. *Comments:*	☐	☐	☐	
4. Follow the five rights of medication administration. *Comments:*	☐	☐	☐	
5. Allow client to manipulate canister. Demonstrate how canister fits into inhaler. Allow client to return demonstrate. *Comments:*	☐	☐	☐	
6. Explain purpose of metered-dose inhaler and purpose of medication, dose, and frequency. *Comments:*	☐	☐	☐	
7. Shake the prepackaged inhaler. Have the client shake the inhaler before each puff. *Comments:*	☐	☐	☐	
8. Place the canister into the applicator. • Place the aerochamber onto the inhaler if needed. *Comments:*	☐	☐	☐	
9. Have the client place the mouthpiece in mouth. *Comments:*	☐	☐	☐	

Procedure 30-11	Able to Perform	Able to Perform with Assistance	Unable to Perform	Initials and Date
10. Have client press down on the dispenser and inhale simultaneously once. • If an aerochamber is used, have the client inhale slowly and deeply. *Comments:*	☐	☐	☐	
11. Have the client remove the mouthpiece and hold breath for 10 seconds, then slowly exhale. *Comments:*	☐	☐	☐	
12. Have the client repeat does as required, waiting one full minute between inhalations. • Have the client wait 5 to 10 minutes before taking other prescribed medications via metered-dose inhaler. *Comments:*	☐	☐	☐	
13. Wash hands. *Comments:*	☐	☐	☐	
14. Record the medication administration and your observations. *Comments:*	☐	☐	☐	
15. Observe client to assess for possible adverse effects. *Comments:*	☐	☐	☐	

_____   _____
Faculty Signature   Date

Checklist for Procedure 30-12 Administering Rectal Medications

Name _____ Date _____

School _____

Instructor _____

Course _____

Procedure 30-12 **Administering Rectal Medications**	Able to Perform	Able to Perform with Assistance	Unable to Perform	Initials and Date
Assessment				
1. Review the order and identify the medication to be delivered. *Comments:*	☐	☐	☐	
2. Assess the client's need for rectal medication administration. *Comments:*	☐	☐	☐	
3. Consider any adjustments needed due to the age of the client. *Comments:*	☐	☐	☐	
4. Observe for the desired effects or any adverse reactions. *Comments:*	☐	☐	☐	
5. Assess the client's understanding of the procedure. *Comments:*	☐	☐	☐	
Planning/Expected Outcomes				
1. The medication will be delivered appropriately and safely. *Comments:*	☐	☐	☐	
2. The desired outcome will be verbalized by the client and documented by the nurse. *Comments:*	☐	☐	☐	
3. The treatment will be completed quickly and efficiently. *Comments:*	☐	☐	☐	
4. Client will state relief of complaint. *Comments:*	☐	☐	☐	

continued on the following page

continued from the previous page

Procedure 30-12	Able to Perform	Able to Perform with Assistance	Unable to Perform	Initials and Date
Implementation				
1. Assess the client's need for the medication. *Comments:*	☐	☐	☐	
2. Check physician or qualified practitioner's written order. *Comments:*	☐	☐	☐	
3. Check the MAR against the medication order. *Comments:*	☐	☐	☐	
4. Check for any drug allergies. *Comments:*	☐	☐	☐	
5. Review the client's history for surgeries or bleeding. *Comments:*	☐	☐	☐	
6. Gather the equipment needed before entering the room. *Comments:*	☐	☐	☐	
7. Assess the client's readiness. Provide privacy. *Comments:*	☐	☐	☐	
8. Wash hands. *Comments:*	☐	☐	☐	
9. Apply disposable gloves. *Comments:*	☐	☐	☐	
10. Ask the client's name and check identification band. *Comments:*	☐	☐	☐	
11. Assist client into correct position. *Comments:*	☐	☐	☐	
12. Visually assess the client's external anus. *Comments:*	☐	☐	☐	
13. Lubricate the enema tip or remove suppository from wrapper and lubricate. *Comments:*	☐	☐	☐	

Procedure 30-12	Able to Perform	Able to Perform with Assistance	Unable to Perform	Initials and Date
14. Explain that client will experience a cool sensation and pressure. *Comments:*	☐	☐	☐	
15. Retract buttocks, visualizing the anus. • Gently insert the suppository through the anus. • Insert the enema tip and instill the contents. *Comments:*	☐	☐	☐	
16. Remove finger or enema tip and clean client's anal area. *Comments:*	☐	☐	☐	
17. Discard gloves. *Comments:*	☐	☐	☐	
18. Wash hands. *Comments:*	☐	☐	☐	
19. Have client remain in bed or on side for 10 minutes. *Comments:*	☐	☐	☐	
20. Place call light within client's reach. *Comments:*	☐	☐	☐	
21. Record administration of medication. *Comments:*	☐	☐	☐	
22. Document effectiveness or any side effects of treatment. *Comments:*	☐	☐	☐	

Faculty Signature

Date

Checklist for Procedure 30-13   Administering Vaginal Medications

Name _____ Date _____

School _____

Instructor _____

Course _____

Procedure 30-13 Administering Vaginal Medications	Able to Perform	Able to Perform with Assistance	Unable to Perform	Initials and Date
Assessment				
1. Assess the client's comfort level and symptoms. *Comments:*	☐	☐	☐	
2. Assess the client's knowledge of the purpose of the treatment. *Comments:*	☐	☐	☐	
3. Assess the client's ability to self-administer the medication. *Comments:*	☐	☐	☐	
Planning/Expected Outcomes				
1. Client will experience an absence of infection. *Comments:*	☐	☐	☐	
2. Client will experience an absence of symptoms. *Comments:*	☐	☐	☐	
3. Client will understand the need to perform the entire course of treatment. *Comments:*	☐	☐	☐	
4. Client will understand the importance of personal hygiene. *Comments:*	☐	☐	☐	
5. Client will understand the need to clean and store equipment. *Comments:*	☐	☐	☐	
Implementation				
1. Verify orders. *Comments:*	☐	☐	☐	

continued on the following page

continued from the previous page

Procedure 30-13	Able to Perform	Able to Perform with Assistance	Unable to Perform	Initials and Date
2. Ascertain that the client understands the procedure. *Comments:*	☐	☐	☐	
3. Ask the client to void. *Comments:*	☐	☐	☐	
4. Wash hands. *Comments:*	☐	☐	☐	
5. Arrange equipment at client's bedside. *Comments:*	☐	☐	☐	
6. Provide privacy. *Comments:*	☐	☐	☐	
7. Assist the client into a dorsal-recumbent or Sim's position. *Comments:*	☐	☐	☐	
8. Drape the client as appropriate. *Comments:*	☐	☐	☐	
9. Position lighting to illuminate vaginal orifice. *Comments:*	☐	☐	☐	
10. Assess the perineal area. *Comments:*	☐	☐	☐	
11. • If using an applicator, fill with medication. • If using a suppository, remove the suppository from the foil and position in the applicator. • Apply water-soluble lubricant to suppository or applicator. *Comments:*	☐	☐	☐	
12. For suppository, retract the labia. *Comments:*	☐	☐	☐	
13. Insert applicator 2 to 3 inches into the vagina. Push the plunger to administer the medication. • Insert the suppository, tapered end first, along the posterior wall of the vagina. *Comments:*	☐	☐	☐	

Procedure 30-13	Able to Perform	Able to Perform with Assistance	Unable to Perform	Initials and Date
14. Withdraw the applicator and place on a towel. *Comments:*	☐	☐	☐	
15. If administering a douche or irrigation: • Warm solution to slightly above body temperature. • Position the client on a bedpan, toilet seat, or in a tub. • Apply lubricant to the irrigation nozzle and insert into the vagina. • Hang the irrigant container approximately 2 feet above the vaginal area. • Open the clamp and allow a small amount of solution to flow into the vagina. • Move the nozzle and rotate around the entire vaginal area. *Comments:*	☐	☐	☐	
16. Wipe and clean the client's perineal area. *Comments:*	☐	☐	☐	
17. Apply a perineal pad. *Comments:*	☐	☐	☐	
18. Wash and store the applicator. *Comments:*	☐	☐	☐	
19. Remove gloves and wash hands. *Comments:*	☐	☐	☐	
20. Instruct the client to remain flat for at least 30 minutes. *Comments:*	☐	☐	☐	
21. Raise side rails and place the call light in reach. *Comments:*	☐	☐	☐	

Faculty Signature

Date

Checklist for Procedure 31-1 Therapeutic Massage

Name _____ Date _____

School _____

Instructor _____

Course _____

Procedure 31-1 **Therapeutic Massage**	Able to Perform	Able to Perform with Assistance	Unable to Perform	Initials and Date
Assessment				
1. Assess the client's current emotional and physical condition. *Comments:*	☐	☐	☐	
2. Review the client's current diagnosis. *Comments:*	☐	☐	☐	
3. Assess the client's current physical surroundings. *Comments:*	☐	☐	☐	
Planning/Expected Outcomes				
1. Client's relaxation will be increased. *Comments:*	☐	☐	☐	
2. Circulation to the massaged area will be increased. *Comments:*	☐	☐	☐	
Implementation				
1. Provide low or indirect lighting, privacy, background music, and a warm room. *Comments:*	☐	☐	☐	
2. Place a clean sheet on the table or bed. Adjust the surface height. *Comments:*	☐	☐	☐	
3. Remove your rings and watches. Wash hands. *Comments:*	☐	☐	☐	
4. Explain the procedure to the client. *Comments:*	☐	☐	☐	
5. Assist the client to a prone, supine, or sitting position. *Comments:*	☐	☐	☐	

continued on the following page

continued from the previous page

Procedure 31-1	Able to Perform	Able to Perform with Assistance	Unable to Perform	Initials and Date
6. Loosen or remove client's clothing. Drape the areas not being treated directly with a sheet. *Comments:*	☐	☐	☐	
7. Warm a small amount of lotion or oil into the palm of the hand. *Comments:*	☐	☐	☐	
8. Begin with light to medium effleurage at lower back and continue upward following muscle groups. Continue the effleurage for approximately 3 minutes. *Comments:*	☐	☐	☐	
9. Continue treatment, if appropriate, with gentle petrissage. *Comments:*	☐	☐	☐	
10. Use friction on particular muscle groups where tension is being held. *Comments:*	☐	☐	☐	
11. Use tapotement to stimulate any muscle groups that may be fatigued. *Comments:*	☐	☐	☐	
12. Finish treatment with effleurage. *Comments:*	☐	☐	☐	
13. Clean any excess lotion or oil from skin with a towel or soap and water. *Comments:*	☐	☐	☐	
14. Assist client into a comfortable position for a period of rest or sleep. *Comments:*	☐	☐	☐	
15. Document treatment. *Comments:*	☐	☐	☐	
16. Wash hands. *Comments:*	☐	☐	☐	

_____   _____

Faculty Signature   Date

Checklist for Procedure 33-1   Applying Restraints

Name _____ Date _____

School _____

Instructor _____

Course _____

Procedure 33-1 **Applying Restraints**	Able to Perform	Able to Perform with Assistance	Unable to Perform	Initials and Date
Assessment				
1. Ensure there is an order or urgent medical need to apply restraints (of any kind) on client. A physician's order is legally required. *Comments:*	☐	☐	☐	
2. Assess the client's level of consciousness. *Comments:*	☐	☐	☐	
3. Assess the client's degree of orientation. *Comments:*	☐	☐	☐	
4. Assess the client's physical condition. *Comments:*	☐	☐	☐	
5. Assess the client's history. *Comments:*	☐	☐	☐	
6. Assess the client's intent. *Comments:*	☐	☐	☐	
7. Assess client's and family's knowledge regarding the use of protective devices. *Comments:*	☐	☐	☐	
Planning/Expected Outcomes				
1. The client will remain uninjured. *Comments:*	☐	☐	☐	
2. The client will not suffer injury or impairment from the restraints. *Comments:*	☐	☐	☐	

                    continued on the following page

continued from the previous page

Procedure 33-1	Able to Perform	Able to Perform with Assistance	Unable to Perform	Initials and Date
3. The client's therapeutic equipment will remain intact and functional. *Comments:*	☐	☐	☐	
4. Others will not be harmed by the client. *Comments:*	☐	☐	☐	
5. The client will be restrained just enough to prevent injury. *Comments:*	☐	☐	☐	

Implementation

Chest Restraint

	Able to Perform	Able to Perform with Assistance	Unable to Perform	Initials and Date
1. Explain that the client will be wearing a jacket attached to the bed for his safety. *Comments:*	☐	☐	☐	
2. Place the restraint over the client's hospital gown or clothing. *Comments:*	☐	☐	☐	
3. Place the restraint with the opening in the front. *Comments:*	☐	☐	☐	
4. Overlap the front pieces, threading the ties through the appropriate slots. *Comments:*	☐	☐	☐	
5. In bed, secure the ties to the movable part of the mattress frame with a half-knot. *Comments:*	☐	☐	☐	
6. In a chair, cross the straps behind the seat and secure to the chair's lower legs. *Comments:*	☐	☐	☐	
7. Step back and assess the client's overall safety. *Comments:*	☐	☐	☐	
8. Wash your hands. *Comments:*	☐	☐	☐	

Procedure 33-1	Able to Perform	Able to Perform with Assistance	Unable to Perform	Initials and Date
Wrist or Ankle Restraints				
1. Explain that you will be placing a wrist or ankle band that will restrict movement. *Comments:*	☐	☐	☐	
2. Place padding around the client's wrist/ankle. *Comments:*	☐	☐	☐	
3. Wrap the restraint around the wrist/ankle, pulling the tie through the appropriate loops. *Comments:*	☐	☐	☐	
4. Tie to the movable portion of the mattress frame with a secure knot. *Comments:*	☐	☐	☐	
5. Slip two fingers under the restraint to check for tightness. *Comments:*	☐	☐	☐	
6. Step back and assess the client's overall safety. *Comments:*	☐	☐	☐	
7. Place the call light within the client's reach. *Comments:*	☐	☐	☐	
8. Check on the client every half hour while restrained. *Comments:*	☐	☐	☐	
9. Assess circulatory status of restrained extremity every 2 hours and as needed. Release one restraint from each extremity for at least 15 minutes every 2 hours and record. *Comments:*	☐	☐	☐	
10. Wash your hands. *Comments:*	☐	☐	☐	

Faculty Signature　　　　　　　　　　　　　　　　Date

Checklist for Procedure 33-2   Bathing a Client in Bed

Name _____   Date _____

School _____

Instructor _____

Course _____

Procedure 33-2 Bathing a Client in Bed	Able to Perform	Able to Perform with Assistance	Unable to Perform	Initials and Date
Assessment				
1. Assess the client's level of ability to assist with the bath. *Comments:*	☐	☐	☐	
2. Assess the client's level of comfort with the procedure. *Comments:*	☐	☐	☐	
3. Assess the environment and equipment available. *Comments:*	☐	☐	☐	
Planning/Expected Outcomes				
1. Client will be cleaned without damage to skin. *Comments:*	☐	☐	☐	
2. Client's privacy will be maintained. *Comments:*	☐	☐	☐	
3. Client will participate in her own hygiene. *Comments:*	☐	☐	☐	
4. Client will not experience adverse effects as a result of the bath. *Comments:*	☐	☐	☐	
Implementation				
1. Assess client's preferences about bathing. *Comments:*	☐	☐	☐	
2. Explain procedure to client. *Comments:*	☐	☐	☐	
3. Prepare environment. Provide time for elimination, and provide privacy. *Comments:*	☐	☐	☐	

     continued on the following page

continued from the previous page

Procedure 33-2	Able to Perform	Able to Perform with Assistance	Unable to Perform	Initials and Date
4. Wash hands. Apply gloves. *Comments:*	☐	☐	☐	
5. Lower side rail nearest you. Position client comfortably. *Comments:*	☐	☐	☐	
6. Place bath blanket over top sheet. Remove top sheet and client's gown. *Comments:*	☐	☐	☐	
7. Fill washbasin two thirds full with warm water. *Comments:*	☐	☐	☐	
8. Wet the washcloth and wring it out. *Comments:*	☐	☐	☐	
9. Make a bath mitten with the washcloth. *Comments:*	☐	☐	☐	
10. Wash client's face, neck, and ears. Shave client if needed. *Comments:*	☐	☐	☐	
11. Wash arms, forearms, and hands. *Comments:*	☐	☐	☐	
12. Wash chest and abdomen. *Comments:*	☐	☐	☐	
13. Wash legs and feet. *Comments:*	☐	☐	☐	
14. Wash back. *Comments:*	☐	☐	☐	
15. Assist client to supine position. Perform perineal care. *Comments:*	☐	☐	☐	
16. Apply lotion and powder as desired. Apply clean gown. *Comments:*	☐	☐	☐	

Procedure 33-2	Able to Perform	Able to Perform with Assistance	Unable to Perform	Initials and Date
17. Document skin assessment, type of bath, and client response. Comments:	☐	☐	☐	
18. Wash hands. Comments:	☐	☐	☐	

_____   _____

Faculty Signature   Date

Checklist for Procedure 33-3   Changing Linens in an Unoccupied Bed

Name _____ Date _____

School _____

Instructor _____

Course _____

Procedure 33-3 Changing Linens in an Unoccupied Bed	Able to Perform	Able to Perform with Assistance	Unable to Perform	Initials and Date
Assessment				
1. Assess your equipment. *Comments:*	☐	☐	☐	
2. Assess whether the bed itself needs cleaning. *Comments:*	☐	☐	☐	
3. Assess the client's needs in the bed. *Comments:*	☐	☐	☐	
Planning/Expected Outcomes				
1. The client will have clean linens on the bed. *Comments:*	☐	☐	☐	
2. The clean linens will be appropriate to the client's needs and condition. *Comments:*	☐	☐	☐	
Implementation				
Preparation 1. Place hamper close by. Explain procedure to client. Assess condition of blankets. *Comments:*	☐	☐	☐	
2. Gather linens and gloves. *Comments:*	☐	☐	☐	
3. Apply gloves. *Comments:*	☐	☐	☐	
4. Attend to the client's needs as necessary. *Comments:*	☐	☐	☐	
5. Assist client to a safe, comfortable chair. *Comments:*	☐	☐	☐	

          continued on the following page

continued from the previous page

Procedure 33-3	Able to Perform	Able to Perform with Assistance	Unable to Perform	Initials and Date
6. Position bed. *Comments:*	☐	☐	☐	
7. Remove and fold blanket and/or bedspread. *Comments:*	☐	☐	☐	
8. Remove soiled pillowcases. *Comments:*	☐	☐	☐	
9. Remove soiled linens. *Comments:*	☐	☐	☐	
10. Fold soiled linens. *Comments:*	☐	☐	☐	
11. Check the mattress. If soiled, clean appropriately. *Comments:*	☐	☐	☐	
12. Remove gloves, wash hands, and apply a second pair of clean gloves. *Comments:*	☐	☐	☐	
13. Place clean mattress pad onto the bed. Unfold half of the pad's width to the center crease. *Comments:*	☐	☐	☐	
14. Proceed with placing bottom sheet onto the mattress. *Comments:*	☐	☐	☐	
Fitted Bottom Sheet 15. Position yourself diagonally toward the head of the bed. *Comments:*	☐	☐	☐	
16. Start at the head with seamed side of the fitted sheet toward the mattress. *Comments:*	☐	☐	☐	
17. Lift the mattress corner and tuck the fitted sheet over the mattress corner. Repeat for other corner. *Comments:*	☐	☐	☐	

Procedure 33-3	Able to Perform	Able to Perform with Assistance	Unable to Perform	Initials and Date
18. Tuck the fitted sheet over the mattress corners at foot of the bed. *Comments:*	☐	☐	☐	
Flat Regular Sheet 19. Align the bottom edge of the sheet with the edge of the mattress at the foot of the bed. *Comments:*	☐	☐	☐	
20. Allow the sheet to hang over the mattress on the side and at the top of the bed. *Comments:*	☐	☐	☐	
21. Position yourself diagonally toward the head of the bed. Lift the mattress corner and smoothly tuck the sheet under the mattress. *Comments:*	☐	☐	☐	
22. Miter the corner at the head of the bed. *Comments:*	☐	☐	☐	
23. Lift and lay the top edge of the sheet onto the bed to form a triangular fold. *Comments:*	☐	☐	☐	
24. Tuck the lower edge of the sheet under the mattress. *Comments:*	☐	☐	☐	
25. Bring the triangular fold down over the side of the mattress. *Comments:*	☐	☐	☐	
26. Place the draw sheet on the bottom sheet and unfold it to the middle crease. *Comments:*	☐	☐	☐	
27. Tuck both the bottom and draw sheets smoothly under the mattress. *Comments:*	☐	☐	☐	
28. On the other side of the bed, repeat steps 13 through 18, as used to apply the mattress pad and bottom sheet. *Comments:*	☐	☐	☐	

                    continued on the following page

continued from the previous page

Procedure 33-3	Able to Perform	Able to Perform with Assistance	Unable to Perform	Initials and Date
29. Unfold the draw sheet and grasp both sheets. Pull toward you and tuck both sheets under the mattress. *Comments:*	☐	☐	☐	
30. Place the top sheet on the bed. Place the top edge of the sheet even with the top of the mattress. Pull the remaining length toward the bottom of the bed. *Comments:*	☐	☐	☐	
31. Unfold and apply the blanket/spread as with the top sheet. *Comments:*	☐	☐	☐	
32. Miter the bottom corners. *Comments:*	☐	☐	☐	
33. Fold the top sheet and blanket over. Fan-fold the sheet and blanket. *Comments:*	☐	☐	☐	
34. Apply clean pillowcase on each pillow. *Comments:*	☐	☐	☐	
35. Place bed in lowest position; raise the head of the bed. *Comments:*	☐	☐	☐	
36. Inquire about toileting needs of the client; assist as necessary. *Comments:*	☐	☐	☐	
37. Assist the client back into the bed and pull up the side rails; place call light in reach; take vital signs. *Comments:*	☐	☐	☐	
38. Remove gloves and wash hands. *Comments:*	☐	☐	☐	
39. Document your actions and the client's response to the activity. *Comments:*	☐	☐	☐	

_____   _____

Faculty Signature   Date

Checklist for Procedure 33-4   Changing Linens in an Occupied Bed

Name _____ Date _____

School _____

Instructor _____

Course _____

Procedure 33-4 Changing Linens in an Occupied Bed	Able to Perform	Able to Perform with Assistance	Unable to Perform	Initials and Date
Assessment				
1. Assess your equipment. *Comments:*	☐	☐	☐	
2. Assess whether the bed itself needs cleaning. *Comments:*	☐	☐	☐	
3. Assess the client's needs in the bed. *Comments:*	☐	☐	☐	
4. Assess the client's ability to assist with the procedure. *Comments:*	☐	☐	☐	
Planning/Expected Outcomes				
1. The client will have clean linens on the bed. *Comments:*	☐	☐	☐	
2. The linens will be appropriate to the client's needs. *Comments:*	☐	☐	☐	
3. The linens will be changed with a minimum of trauma to the client. *Comments:*	☐	☐	☐	
Implementation				
1. Explain procedure to client. *Comments:*	☐	☐	☐	
2. Bring equipment to the bedside. *Comments:*	☐	☐	☐	
3. Remove top sheet and blanket. Loosen bottom sheet. *Comments:*	☐	☐	☐	
4. Position client on side, facing away from you. *Comments:*	☐	☐	☐	

continued on the following page

continued from the previous page

Procedure 33-4	Able to Perform	Able to Perform with Assistance	Unable to Perform	Initials and Date
5. Fan-fold or roll bottom linens toward the center of the bed. *Comments:*	☐	☐	☐	
6. Place clean bottom linens. Fan-fold or roll clean bottom linens and tuck under soiled linen. *Comments:*	☐	☐	☐	
7. Miter bottom sheet at head and foot of bed. Tuck the sides of the sheet under the mattress. *Comments:*	☐	☐	☐	
8. Fan-fold or roll draw sheet and tuck under soiled linen. Tuck draw sheet under mattress. *Comments:*	☐	☐	☐	
9. Log roll client over onto side facing you. Raise side rail. *Comments:*	☐	☐	☐	
10. At the other side of bed, remove soiled linens. *Comments:*	☐	☐	☐	
11. Unfold/unroll bottom sheet; then draw sheet. Tuck in. *Comments:*	☐	☐	☐	
12. Place top sheet and blanket over client. *Comments:*	☐	☐	☐	
13. Raise foot of mattress and miter the corner. Repeat on other side. *Comments:*	☐	☐	☐	
14. Tent top sheet and blanket over client's toes. *Comments:*	☐	☐	☐	
15. Remove and replace pillowcase. *Comments:*	☐	☐	☐	
16. Document procedure and client's condition. *Comments:*	☐	☐	☐	
17. Wash hands. *Comments:*	☐	☐	☐	

Faculty Signature   Date

Checklist for Procedure 33-5　Perineal and Genital Care

Name _____ Date _____

School _____

Instructor _____

Course _____

Procedure 33-5 **Perineal and Genital Care**	Able to Perform	Able to Perform with Assistance	Unable to Perform	Initials and Date
Assessment				
1. Evaluate client status. *Comments:*	☐	☐	☐	
2. Identify cultural preferences for perineal care. *Comments:*	☐	☐	☐	
3. Assess the client's perineal health. *Comments:*	☐	☐	☐	
4. Determine if the client is incontinent of urine or stool. *Comments:*				
5. Assess whether the client has recently had perineal/genital surgery. *Comments:*	☐	☐	☐	
Planning/Expected Outcomes				
1. Perineum and genitalia will be dry, clean, and odor free. *Comments:*	☐	☐	☐	
2. The client will report feeling comfortable and clean. *Comments:*	☐	☐	☐	
3. The client will not experience discomfort or undue embarrassment. *Comments:*	☐	☐	☐	
4. The perineum will be free of skin breakdown or irritation. *Comments:*	☐	☐	☐	

　　　　continued on the following page

continued from the previous page

Procedure 33-5	Able to Perform	Able to Perform with Assistance	Unable to Perform	Initials and Date
Implementation				
1. Wash hands and wear gloves. *Comments:*	☐	☐	☐	
2. Close privacy curtain or door. *Comments:*	☐	☐	☐	
3. Position client. *Comments:*	☐	☐	☐	
4. Place waterproof pads under the client. *Comments:*	☐	☐	☐	
5. Remove fecal debris and dispose in toilet. *Comments:*	☐	☐	☐	
6. Spray perineum with washing solution. *Comments:*	☐	☐	☐	
7. Cleanse perineum with wet washcloths. Cleanse the penis on the male. *Comments:*	☐	☐	☐	
8. Examine folds and vulva for debris. *Comments:*	☐	☐	☐	
9. If soap is used, spray area with clean water from the peri-bottle. *Comments:*	☐	☐	☐	
10. Change gloves. *Comments:*	☐	☐	☐	
11. Dry perineum carefully with towel. *Comments:*	☐	☐	☐	
12. If indicated, apply barrier lotion or ointment. *Comments:*	☐	☐	☐	

Procedure 33-5	Able to Perform	Able to Perform with Assistance	Unable to Perform	Initials and Date
13. Reposition or dress client as appropriate. *Comments:*	☐	☐	☐	
14. Dispose of linens and garbage appropriately. *Comments:*	☐	☐	☐	
15. Wash hands. *Comments:*	☐	☐	☐	
16. Deodorize room if appropriate. *Comments:*	☐	☐	☐	

_____   _____

Faculty Signature   Date

Checklist for Procedure 33-6   Oral Care

Name _____ Date _____

School _____

Instructor _____

Course _____

Procedure 33-6 Oral Care	Able to Perform	Able to Perform with Assistance	Unable to Perform	Initials and Date
Assessment				
1. Assess whether the client is able to assist with oral care. *Comments:*	☐	☐	☐	
2. Evaluate whether the client has an understanding of proper oral hygiene. *Comments:*	☐	☐	☐	
3. Determine whether the client has dentures. *Comments:*	☐	☐	☐	
4. Assess the condition of the client's mouth. *Comments:*	☐	☐	☐	
5. Assess mouth for disease processes. *Comments:*	☐	☐	☐	
6. Assess what cultural practices must be considered. *Comments:*	☐	☐	☐	
7. Assess whether there are any appliances or devices present in the client's mouth. *Comments:*	☐	☐	☐	
8. Ensure that the proper equipment is available. *Comments:*	☐	☐	☐	
Planning/Expected Outcomes				
1. Client's mouth, teeth, gums, and lips will be clean. *Comments:*	☐	☐	☐	
2. Any disease processes present will be noted and treated. *Comments:*	☐	☐	☐	

                    continued on the following page

continued from the previous page

Procedure 33-6	Able to Perform	Able to Perform with Assistance	Unable to Perform	Initials and Date
3. The oral mucosa will be clean, intact, and well hydrated. *Comments:*	☐	☐	☐	

Implementation

Self-Care Client: Flossing and Brushing

1. Assemble articles for flossing and brushing. *Comments:*	☐	☐	☐	
2. Provide privacy. *Comments:*	☐	☐	☐	
3. Place client in a high-Fowler's position. *Comments:*	☐	☐	☐	
4. Wash hands and apply gloves. *Comments:*	☐	☐	☐	
5. Arrange articles within client's reach. *Comments:*	☐	☐	☐	
6. Assist client with flossing and brushing as necessary. *Comments:*	☐	☐	☐	
7. Assist client with rinsing mouth. *Comments:*	☐	☐	☐	
8. Reposition client, raise side rails, and place call button within reach. *Comments:*	☐	☐	☐	
9. Rinse, dry, and return articles to proper place. *Comments:*	☐	☐	☐	
10. Remove gloves, wash hands, and document care. *Comments:*	☐	☐	☐	

Self-Care Client: Denture Care

11. Assemble articles for denture cleaning. *Comments:*	☐	☐	☐	

Procedure 33-6	Able to Perform	Able to Perform with Assistance	Unable to Perform	Initials and Date
12. Provide privacy. *Comments:*	☐	☐	☐	
13. Assist client to a high-Fowler's position. *Comments:*	☐	☐	☐	
14. Wash hands and apply gloves. *Comments:*	☐	☐	☐	
15. Assist client with denture removal. Place in denture cup. *Comments:*	☐	☐	☐	
16. Apply toothpaste to brush and brush dentures with cool water. If brushing dentures at the client's sink, place a washcloth in the sink basin to prevent breaking dentures if they are dropped. *Comments:*	☐	☐	☐	
17. Rinse dentures thoroughly. *Comments:*	☐	☐	☐	
18. Assist client with rinsing mouth and replacing dentures. *Comments:*	☐	☐	☐	
19. Reposition client, with side rails up and call button within reach. *Comments:*	☐	☐	☐	
20. Rinse, dry, and return articles to proper place. *Comments:*	☐	☐	☐	
21. Remove gloves, wash hands, and document care. *Comments:*	☐	☐	☐	
Full-Care Client: Brushing and Flossing 22. Assemble articles for flossing and brushing. *Comments:*	☐	☐	☐	
23. Provide privacy. *Comments:*	☐	☐	☐	

                    continued on the following page

continued from the previous page

Procedure 33-6	Able to Perform	Able to Perform with Assistance	Unable to Perform	Initials and Date
24. Wash hands and apply gloves. *Comments:*	☐	☐	☐	
25. Position client as condition allows. *Comments:*	☐	☐	☐	
26. Place towel across client's chest or under face and mouth. *Comments:*	☐	☐	☐	
27. Apply small amount of toothpaste, and brush teeth and gums. *Comments:*	☐	☐	☐	
28. Floss between all teeth. *Comments:*	☐	☐	☐	
29. Assist the client in rinsing mouth. *Comments:*	☐	☐	☐	
30. Reapply toothpaste and brush the teeth and gums. *Comments:*	☐	☐	☐	
31. Assist the client in rinsing and drying mouth. *Comments:*	☐	☐	☐	
32. Apply lip moisturizer, if appropriate. *Comments:*	☐	☐	☐	
33. Reposition client, raise side rails, and place call button within reach. *Comments:*	☐	☐	☐	
34. Rinse, dry, and return articles to proper place. *Comments:*	☐	☐	☐	
35. Remove gloves, wash hands, and document care. *Comments:*	☐	☐	☐	

Procedure 33-6	Able to Perform	Able to Perform with Assistance	Unable to Perform	Initials and Date
Clients at Risk for or with an Alteration of the Oral Cavity				
36. Assemble articles for flossing and brushing. *Comments:*	☐	☐	☐	
37. Provide privacy. *Comments:*	☐	☐	☐	
38. Wash hands and apply gloves. *Comments:*	☐	☐	☐	

39. Bleeding:
   a. Assess oral cavity for signs of bleeding.
   b. Proceed with the oral care for a full-care client, except:
     • Do not floss.
     • Use a soft toothbrush, toothette, or a padded tongue blade to swab teeth and gums.
     • Dispose of padded tongue blade into a biohazard bag.
     • Rinse with tepid water.
 Comments:
	☐	☐	☐	

40. Infection:
   a. Assess oral cavity for signs of infection.
   b. Culture lesions as ordered.
   c. Proceed with oral care for a full-care client except:
     • Do not floss.
     • Use prescribed antiseptic solution.
     • Use a padded tongue blade to swab the teeth and gums.
     • Dispose of padded tongue blade into a biohazard bag.
     • Rinse mouth with tepid water.
     • Apply additional solution as prescribed.
 Comments:
	☐	☐	☐	

41. Ulceration:
   a. Assess oral cavity for signs of ulceration.
   b. Culture lesions as ordered.
   c. Proceed with oral care for a full-care client except:
     • Do not floss.
     • Use prescribed antiseptic solution.
     • Use a padded tongue blade to swab the teeth and gums.
     • Dispose of padded tongue blade into a biohazard bag.
     • Rinse mouth with tepid water.
     • Apply additional solution as prescribed.
 Comments:
	☐	☐	☐	

                    continued on the following page

continued from the previous page

Procedure 33-6	Able to Perform	Able to Perform with Assistance	Unable to Perform	Initials and Date
Unconscious (Comatose) Client:				
42. Assemble articles for flossing and brushing. *Comments:*	☐	☐	☐	
43. Provide privacy. *Comments:*	☐	☐	☐	
44. Wash hands and apply gloves. *Comments:*	☐	☐	☐	
45. Explain the procedure to the client. *Comments:*	☐	☐	☐	
46. Place the client in a lateral position, head turned toward the side. *Comments:*	☐	☐	☐	
47. Use a floss holder and floss between all teeth. *Comments:*	☐	☐	☐	
48. Moisten toothbrush, and brush the teeth and gums. Do not use toothpaste. *Comments:*	☐	☐	☐	
49. After flossing and brushing, rinse mouth and perform oral suction. *Comments:*	☐	☐	☐	
50. Dry the client's mouth. *Comments:*	☐	☐	☐	
51. Apply lip moisturizer. *Comments:*	☐	☐	☐	
52. Leave the client in a lateral position for 30 to 60 minutes after oral care. Suction one more time. *Comments:*	☐	☐	☐	
53. Dispose of nonreusable items appropriately. Rinse, dry, and return articles to proper place. *Comments:*	☐	☐	☐	
54. Remove gloves, wash hands, and document care. *Comments:*	☐	☐	☐	

_____   _____

Faculty Signature   Date

Checklist for Procedure 33-7   Eye Care

Name _____   Date _____

School _____

Instructor _____

Course _____

Procedure 33-7 Eye Care	Able to Perform	Able to Perform with Assistance	Unable to Perform	Initials and Date
Assessment				
1. Determine if the client is wearing contact lenses or has an ocular prosthesis. *Comments:*	☐	☐	☐	
2. Determine availability of eye care supplies. *Comments:*	☐	☐	☐	
3. Assess whether the client can do his own eye care. *Comments:*	☐	☐	☐	
Planning/Expected Outcomes				
1. The client's contact lenses will be safely removed and stored. *Comments:*	☐	☐	☐	
2. The client's ocular prosthesis will be safely removed, cleaned, and either stored or returned to the client's eye socket. *Comments:*	☐	☐	☐	
3. The client's contacts or prosthesis will be cared for with a minimum of trauma to the client. *Comments:*	☐	☐	☐	
4. The client's eyes will be free of crusts and exudate. *Comments:*	☐	☐	☐	
Implementation				
Artificial Eye Removal 1. Inquire about client's care regimen and gather equipment. *Comments:*	☐	☐	☐	
2. Provide privacy. *Comments:*	☐	☐	☐	

                    continued on the following page

continued from the previous page

Procedure 33-7	Able to Perform	Able to Perform with Assistance	Unable to Perform	Initials and Date
3. Wash hands; apply gloves. *Comments:*	☐	☐	☐	
4. Place client in a semi-Fowler's position. *Comments:*	☐	☐	☐	
5. Place cotton balls in emesis basin filled halfway with warm water. *Comments:*	☐	☐	☐	
6. Place gauze sponges in bottom of second emesis basin filled halfway with mild soap and tepid water. *Comments:*	☐	☐	☐	
7. Squeeze excess water from a cotton ball. Cleanse the eyelid with the cotton ball. Repeat until eyelid is clean. *Comments:*	☐	☐	☐	
8. Remove the artificial eye. • Raise the client's upper eyelid and depress the lower eyelid. • Cup hand under the client's lower eyelid. • Apply slight pressure between the brow and the artificial eye and remove it. Place it in the warm, soapy water. *Comments:*	☐	☐	☐	
9. With a moistened cotton ball, cleanse the edge of the eye socket. *Comments:*	☐	☐	☐	
10. Inspect the eye socket for irritation, drainage, or crusting. *Comments:*	☐	☐	☐	
11. If irrigation is ordered: • Place the client in flat, supine position. Turn head toward socket side and slightly extend neck. • Fill the irrigation syringe with the irrigating solution. • Separate the eyelids, resting fingers on the brow and cheekbone. • Hold the irrigating syringe several inches above the inner canthus. Direct the flow of solution from the inner canthus along the conjunctival sac. • Irrigate with the prescribed amount of solution.				

Procedure 33-7	Able to Perform	Able to Perform with Assistance	Unable to Perform	Initials and Date
• Wipe the eyelids with a moistened cotton ball. • Pat the skin dry with the towel. • Return the client to a semi-Fowler's position. • Remove gloves, wash hands, and apply clean gloves. *Comments:*	☐	☐	☐	
12. Rub the artificial eye between the fingers in warm, soapy water. *Comments:*	☐	☐	☐	
13. Rinse the prosthesis under running water or in the basin of tepid water. Do not dry the prosthesis. *Comments:*	☐	☐	☐	
14. Reinsert the prosthesis. • With the thumb, raise and hold the upper eyelid open. • Grasp the artificial eye so that the indented part is facing the client's nose and slide it under the upper eyelid. • Depress the lower lid. • Pull the lower lid forward to cover the edge of the prosthesis. *Comments:*	☐	☐	☐	
15. Store prosthesis. • Place the cleaned eye in a labeled container with saline or tap water. *Comments:*	☐	☐	☐	
16. With a moistened cotton ball, wipe the eyelid from the inner to the outer canthus. *Comments:*	☐	☐	☐	
17. Clean, dry, and replace equipment. *Comments:*	☐	☐	☐	
18. Reposition the client, raise side rails, and place call light within reach. *Comments:*	☐	☐	☐	
19. Dispose of biohazard bag appropriately. *Comments:*	☐	☐	☐	

        continued on the following page

continued from the previous page

Procedure 33-7	Able to Perform	Able to Perform with Assistance	Unable to Perform	Initials and Date
20. Remove gloves and wash hands. *Comments:*	☐	☐	☐	
21. Document procedure, client's response, and client teaching. *Comments:*	☐	☐	☐	
Contact Lens Removal 22. Assemble equipment for lens removal. *Comments:*	☐	☐	☐	
23. Assess level of assistance needed, provide privacy, and explain procedure to the client. *Comments:*	☐	☐	☐	
24. Wash hands. *Comments:*	☐	☐	☐	
25. Assist the client to a semi-Fowler's position if needed. *Comments:*	☐	☐	☐	
26. Drape a clean towel over the client's chest. *Comments:*	☐	☐	☐	
27. Prepare the lens storage case with the prescribed solution. *Comments:*	☐	☐	☐	
28. Instruct the client to look straight ahead. Assess the location of the lens. Move the lens toward the cornea. *Comments:*	☐	☐	☐	

29. Remove the lens.
  a. Hard lens:
    • Cup nondominant hand under the eye.
    • Pull outside corner of the eye toward the temple and ask client to blink. Catch the lens.
  b. Soft lens:
    • Separate the eyelid with your fingers.
    • Slide the lens downward onto the sclera and gently squeeze the lens.
    • Release the top eyelid and remove the lens.
    • If lens cannot be extracted using fingers, secure a suction cup to remove the contact lens.
Comments:
	☐	☐	☐	

Procedure 33-7	Able to Perform	Able to Perform with Assistance	Unable to Perform	Initials and Date
30. Store the lens in the correct compartment of a case labeled with the client's name. *Comments:*	☐	☐	☐	
31. Repeat steps 29 and 30 for the second lens. *Comments:*	☐	☐	☐	
32. Assess eyes for irritation or redness. *Comments:*	☐	☐	☐	
33. Store the lens case in a safe place. *Comments:*	☐	☐	☐	
34. Dispose of soiled articles and clean and return reusable articles. *Comments:*	☐	☐	☐	
35. Reposition the client, raise side rails, and place call light within reach. *Comments:*	☐	☐	☐	
36. Remove gloves and wash hands. *Comments:*	☐	☐	☐	
37. Document procedure. *Comments:*	☐	☐	☐	

_____   _____
Faculty Signature   Date

Checklist for Procedure 34-1   Measuring Intake and Output

Name _____ Date _____

School _____

Instructor _____

Course _____

Procedure 34-1 Measuring Intake and Output	Able to Perform	Able to Perform with Assistance	Unable to Perform	Initials and Date
Assessment				
1. Assess the client's risk factors for fluid overload. *Comments:*	☐	☐	☐	
2. Determine if the client is receiving fluids or medications that would predispose her to fluid overload. *Comments:*	☐	☐	☐	
3. Assess the client's risk factors for fluid loss. *Comments:*	☐	☐	☐	
4. Determine if the client's urine output is in excess of her fluid intake. *Comments:*	☐	☐	☐	
5. Assess the client's ability to understand and cooperate with intake and output measurement. *Comments:*	☐	☐	☐	
Planning/Expected Outcomes				
1. The client's fluid intake and output will be accurately measured and recorded. *Comments:*	☐	☐	☐	
2. The client will participate in the recording of fluid intake and output to the best of her ability. *Comments:*	☐	☐	☐	
Implementation				
Intake 1. Wash hands. *Comments:*	☐	☐	☐	

continued on the following page

continued from the previous page

Procedure 34-1	Able to Perform	Able to Perform with Assistance	Unable to Perform	Initials and Date
2. Explain rules of intake and output (I&O) record. *Comments:*	☐	☐	☐	
3. Measure all oral fluids in accord with agency policy. Record all IV fluids as they are infused. *Comments:*	☐	☐	☐	
4. Record time and amount of all fluid intake in the designated space on bedside form. *Comments:*	☐	☐	☐	
5. Transfer 8-hour total fluid intake from bedside I&O record to graphic sheet or 24-hour I&O record on client's chart. *Comments:*	☐	☐	☐	
6. Record all forms of intake, except blood and blood products, in the appropriate column. *Comments:*	☐	☐	☐	
7. Complete 24-hour intake record by adding all 8-hour totals. *Comments:*	☐	☐	☐	
Output 8. Apply nonsterile gloves. *Comments:*	☐	☐	☐	
9. Empty urinal, bedpan, or Foley drainage bag into graduated container or commode "hat." Other output may also be recorded, including nasogastric suction, suction bulb (e.g., Jackson-Pratt or Hemovac), or chest tubes. Refer to agency policy. *Comments:*	☐	☐	☐	
10. Remove gloves and wash hands. *Comments:*	☐	☐	☐	
11. Record time and amount of output on bedside I&O record. *Comments:*	☐	☐	☐	

Procedure 34-1	Able to Perform	Able to Perform with Assistance	Unable to Perform	Initials and Date
12. Transfer 8-hour output totals to graphic sheet or 24-hour I&O record on the client's chart. *Comments:*	☐	☐	☐	
13. Complete 24-hour output record by totaling all 8-hour totals. *Comments:*	☐	☐	☐	
14. Wash hands. *Comments:*	☐	☐	☐	

_____

Faculty Signature

_____

Date

Checklist for Procedure 34-2   Preparing an IV Solution

Name _____ Date _____

School _____

Instructor _____

Course _____

Procedure 34-2 **Preparing an IV Solution**	Able to Perform	Able to Perform with Assistance	Unable to Perform	Initials and Date
Assessment				
1. Check the order for the IV solution and infusion rate. *Comments:*	☐	☐	☐	
2. Review information regarding the solution and nursing implications. *Comments:*	☐	☐	☐	
3. Check all additives in the solution and other medications. *Comments:*	☐	☐	☐	
4. Assess the client's understanding of the purpose of the IV infusion. *Comments:*	☐	☐	☐	
Planning/Expected Outcomes				
1. The appropriate fluids at the ordered dosages will be available. *Comments:*	☐	☐	☐	
2. The IV infusion will be sterile, without precipitate or contamination. *Comments:*	☐	☐	☐	
3. The caregiver preparing the IV solution will not be endangered. *Comments:*	☐	☐	☐	
Implementation				
1. Check the order for the IV solution. *Comments:*	☐	☐	☐	

                         continued on the following page

continued from the previous page

Procedure 34-2	Able to Perform	Able to Perform with Assistance	Unable to Perform	Initials and Date
2. Wash hands. Apply gloves if needed. *Comments:*	☐	☐	☐	
3. Remove protective cover from bag or bottle. *Comments:*	☐	☐	☐	
4. Inspect the bag or bottle. Inspect the fluid. Check expiration date. *Comments:*	☐	☐	☐	
5. Prepare a label for the IV bag or bottle. • Mark date, time, and your initials. • Note the rate at which the solution is to infuse. • Mark approximate infusion intervals on the label. • Attach the label to the bag or bottle upside-down. *Comments:*	☐	☐	☐	
6. Store the prepared IV solution in the assigned area. *Comments:*	☐	☐	☐	
7. Remove gloves and dispose with all used materials. *Comments:*	☐	☐	☐	
8. Wash hands. *Comments:*	☐	☐	☐	
9. Document the preparation of the IV solution. *Comments:*	☐	☐	☐	
Hanging the Prepared IV 10. Wash hands. *Comments:*	☐	☐	☐	
11. Obtain the ordered IV solution. Check to be sure it matches the order. *Comments:*	☐	☐	☐	
12. Inspect the bag or bottle. Inspect the fluid. *Comments:*	☐	☐	☐	

Procedure 34-2	Able to Perform	Able to Perform with Assistance	Unable to Perform	Initials and Date
13. Check client's identification bracelet. *Comments:*	☐	☐	☐	
14. Prepare an IV time tap, noting the IV rate and approximate infusion intervals. Attach tape to solution upside-down. *Comments:*	☐	☐	☐	
15. With the tubing clamp closed, remove the plastic covering from the infusion port and insert the tubing spike into the port. *Comments:*	☐	☐	☐	
16. Compress the drip chamber to fill halfway. *Comments:*	☐	☐	☐	
17. Loosen protective cap from end of tubing, open the roller clamp, and flush tubing with IV solution. *Comments:*	☐	☐	☐	
18. Close the roller clamp and tighten the cap protector. *Comments:*	☐	☐	☐	
19. When ready to initiate the infusion, remove the cap protector and attach the tubing to the IV catheter. *Comments:*	☐	☐	☐	
20. Open the clamp and regulate the flow of solution. *Comments:*	☐	☐	☐	
21. Wash hands. *Comments:*	☐	☐	☐	

_____   _____
Faculty Signature   Date

Checklist for Procedure 34-3 Adding Medications to an IV Solution

Name _____ Date _____

School _____

Instructor _____

Course _____

Procedure 34-3 Adding Medications to an IV Solution	Able to Perform	Able to Perform with Assistance	Unable to Perform	Initials and Date
Assessment				
1. Check the order for the client, medication, dosage, time, and route of administration. *Comments:*	☐	☐	☐	
2. Review information regarding the drug. *Comments:*	☐	☐	☐	
3. Determine the additives in the solution of an existing IV line. *Comments:*	☐	☐	☐	
4. Assess the patency of the IV. *Comments:*	☐	☐	☐	
5. Assess the skin at the IV site. *Comments:*	☐	☐	☐	
6. Assess the client's drug allergy history. *Comments:*	☐	☐	☐	
7. Assess the client's understanding of the purpose of the medication. *Comments:*	☐	☐	☐	
Planning/Expected Outcomes				
1. The appropriate fluids and medications at the ordered dosages will be mixed for IV infusion. *Comments:*	☐	☐	☐	
2. The IV infusion will not be contaminated during the procedure. *Comments:*	☐	☐	☐	

    continued on the following page

continued from the previous page

Procedure 34-3	Able to Perform	Able to Perform with Assistance	Unable to Perform	Initials and Date
3. The caregiver mixing the IV will not be endangered. *Comments:*	☐	☐	☐	
4. The medication will be infused without trauma to the client. *Comments:*	☐	☐	☐	
Implementation				
1. Check order for the IV solution and additives ordered. *Comments:*	☐	☐	☐	
2. Determine whether the ordered additives are compatible with the IV solution and with each other. *Comments:*	☐	☐	☐	
3. Wash hands; apply gloves, if needed. *Comments:*	☐	☐	☐	
4. Using the appropriate technique, draw up ordered additives. *Comments:*	☐	☐	☐	
Adding Medication to a New Solution 5. Remove protective cover from new bag or bottle. *Comments:*	☐	☐	☐	
6. Inspect the bag or bottle. Inspect the fluid. Check expiration date. *Comments:*	☐	☐	☐	
7. Add medication to IV solution. • For plastic IV bag, locate port with rubber stopper. • For IV bottle, locate the X, circle, or triangle over the IV injection site. • Wipe off port or site with antiseptic swab. • Insert needle into center of port or site. • Inject medication into bag. • Remove needle from bag. *Comments:*	☐	☐	☐	
8. Mix medication into IV solution. *Comments:*	☐	☐	☐	

Procedure 34-3	Able to Perform	Able to Perform with Assistance	Unable to Perform	Initials and Date
9. Label the bag. • Write the name and dose of medication, date, time, and your initials. • Apply to bag upside-down. *Comments:*	☐	☐	☐	
10. Store the prepared IV solution in the assigned area. *Comments:*	☐	☐	☐	
Adding Medication to an Existing Solution 11. Identify client by using armband and calling name. *Comments:*	☐	☐	☐	
12. Explain the purpose and route of the medication. *Comments:*	☐	☐	☐	
13. Clamp the IV tubing and remove bag from IV pole. *Comments:*	☐	☐	☐	
14. Add medication to IV solution. • For plastic IV bag, locate port with rubber stopper. • For IV bottle, locate the X, circle, or triangle over the IV injection site. • Wipe off port or site with antiseptic swab. • Insert needle into center of port or site. • Inject medication into bag. • Remove needle from bag. *Comments:*	☐	☐	☐	
15. Mix medication into IV solution. *Comments:*	☐	☐	☐	
16. Apply a new label. • Write the name and dose of medication, date, time, and your initials. • Apply to bag upside-down. *Comments:*	☐	☐	☐	
17. Unclamp the tubing and regulate the flow. *Comments:*	☐	☐	☐	
18. Remove gloves and dispose of all used materials appropriately. *Comments:*	☐	☐	☐	

 continued on the following page

continued from the previous page

Procedure 34-3	Able to Perform	Able to Perform with Assistance	Unable to Perform	Initials and Date
19. Wash hands. *Comments:*	☐	☐	☐	
20. Document the preparation of the IV solution. *Comments:*	☐	☐	☐	

_____   _____

Faculty Signature   Date

Checklist for Procedure 34-4   Assessing and Maintaining an IV Insertion Site

Name _____ Date _____

School _____

Instructor _____

Course _____

Procedure 34-4 **Assessing and Maintaining an IV Insertion Site**	Able to Perform	Able to Perform with Assistance	Unable to Perform	Initials and Date
Assessment				
1. Review the order for IV therapy. *Comments:*	☐	☐	☐	
2. Identify potential risk factors for fluid and electrolyte imbalances. *Comments:*	☐	☐	☐	
3. Assess for dehydration. *Comments:*	☐	☐	☐	
4. Assess for fluid overload. *Comments:*	☐	☐	☐	
5. Determine the client's risk for complications from IV therapy. *Comments:*	☐	☐	☐	
6. Observe IV site for complications. *Comments:*	☐	☐	☐	
7. Observe IV site for patency. *Comments:*	☐	☐	☐	
8. Assess the client's knowledge regarding the IV therapy. *Comments:*	☐	☐	☐	
Planning/Expected Outcomes				
1. The IV will be patent, without infection or inflammation. *Comments:*	☐	☐	☐	
2. The fluid and electrolyte balance will return to and remain normal. *Comments:*	☐	☐	☐	

   continued on the following page

continued from the previous page

Procedure 34-4	Able to Perform	Able to Perform with Assistance	Unable to Perform	Initials and Date
3. The client will be able to report signs of inflammation or infiltration. *Comments:*	☐	☐	☐	
4. The client's IV will be administered per order. *Comments:*	☐	☐	☐	
5. The client's IV dressing will remain intact, clean, and dry. *Comments:*	☐	☐	☐	
Implementation				
1. Review the written order for IV therapy. *Comments:*	☐	☐	☐	
2. Review client's history for medical conditions or allergies. *Comments:*	☐	☐	☐	
3. Review client's IV site record and intake and output record. *Comments:*	☐	☐	☐	
4. Wash hands. *Comments:*	☐	☐	☐	
5. Obtain client's vital signs. *Comments:*	☐	☐	☐	
6. Check IV for correct fluid, additives, rate, and volume at the beginning of your shift. *Comments:*	☐	☐	☐	
7. Check IV tubing for tight connections every 4 hours. *Comments:*	☐	☐	☐	
8. Check gauze IV dressing hourly to be sure it is dry and intact. *Comments:*	☐	☐	☐	
9. If gauze is not dry and intact, observe site for redness, swelling, or drainage every hour. *Comments:*	☐	☐	☐	

Procedure 34-4	Able to Perform	Able to Perform with Assistance	Unable to Perform	Initials and Date
10. If an occlusive dressing is used, do not remove dressing when assessing the site. *Comments:*	☐	☐	☐	
11. Observe vein track hourly. *Comments:*	☐	☐	☐	
12. Document findings in the nursing record or IV flow sheet. *Comments:*	☐	☐	☐	
13. Wash hands. *Comments:*	☐	☐	☐	

Faculty Signature

Date

Checklist for Procedure 34-5 Administering a Blood Transfusion

Name _____ Date _____

School _____

Instructor _____

Course _____

Procedure 34-5 **Administering a Blood Transfusion**	Able to Perform	Able to Perform with Assistance	Unable to Perform	Initials and Date
Assessment				
1. Assess the client for indications requiring the blood product to be given. *Comments:*	☐	☐	☐	
2. Verify the written order for the blood product to be given. *Comments:*	☐	☐	☐	
3. Review the client's transfusion history. *Comments:*	☐	☐	☐	
4. Review the client's baseline vital signs. *Comments:*	☐	☐	☐	
5. Assess the type, integrity, and patency of venous access. *Comments:*	☐	☐	☐	
6. Verify that a large-bore IV catheter is to be used. *Comments:*	☐	☐	☐	
7. Review hospital policy and procedure for the administration of blood products. *Comments:*	☐	☐	☐	
Planning/Expected Outcomes				
1. The client receives the transfusion without adverse reactions or with successfully managed reactions. *Comments:*	☐	☐	☐	
2. The client demonstrates desired benefit from transfusion. *Comments:*	☐	☐	☐	
3. The client understands the purpose and procedure of the transfusion. *Comments:*	☐	☐	☐	

          continued on the following page

continued from the previous page

Procedure 34-5	Able to Perform	Able to Perform with Assistance	Unable to Perform	Initials and Date
4. The client describes the possible complications of a transfusion. *Comments:*	☐	☐	☐	

Implementation

	Able to Perform	Able to Perform with Assistance	Unable to Perform	Initials and Date
1. Verify the written order for the transfusion. *Comments:*	☐	☐	☐	
2. If a venipuncture is necessary, refer to Procedure 29-1 on page 39. *Comments:*	☐	☐	☐	
3. Explain procedure to the client. *Comments:*	☐	☐	☐	
4. Start IV if necessary. *Comments:*	☐	☐	☐	
5. Review side effects with client and have the client report any to the nurse. *Comments:*	☐	☐	☐	
6. Have the client sign consent forms. *Comments:*	☐	☐	☐	
7. Obtain baseline vital signs. *Comments:*	☐	☐	☐	
8. Obtain the blood product from the blood bank within 30 minutes of initiation. *Comments:*	☐	☐	☐	
9. Verify the blood product and the client with another nurse. • Client's name, blood group, Rh type • Cross-match compatibility • Donor blood group and Rh type • Unit and hospital number • Expiration date and time on blood bag • Type of blood product compared with written order • Presence of clots in blood *Comments:*	☐	☐	☐	

Procedure 34-5	Able to Perform	Able to Perform with Assistance	Unable to Perform	Initials and Date
10. Instruct client to empty bladder. *Comments:*	☐	☐	☐	
11. Wash hands and put on gloves. *Comments:*	☐	☐	☐	
12. Open blood administration kit and close roller clamps. *Comments:*	☐	☐	☐	
13. For Y-tubing set: • Spike the normal saline bag and prime the tubing between the saline bag and the filter. • Squeeze sides of drip chamber and allow filter to partially fill. • Open lower roller clamp and prime tubing to the hub. • Close lower clamp. • Invert blood bag once or twice. Spike blood bag, open clamps, and fill tubing completely, covering the filter with blood. • Close lower clamp. *Comments:*	☐	☐	☐	
14. For single-tubing set: • Spike blood unit using filter tubing. • Squeeze drip chamber and allow the filter to fill with blood. • Open roller clamp and allow tubing to fill with blood. • Piggyback a saline line into the blood administration tubing. • Secure all connections with tape. *Comments:*	☐	☐	☐	
15. Attach tubing to venous catheter aseptically and open clamps on blood tubing. *Comments:*	☐	☐	☐	
16. Infuse the blood product at the ordered rate. *Comments:*	☐	☐	☐	
17. Remain with client for first 15 to 30 minutes, monitoring vital signs frequently according to institutional policy. *Comments:*	☐	☐	☐	

          continued on the following page

continued from the previous page

Procedure 34-5	Able to Perform	Able to Perform with Assistance	Unable to Perform	Initials and Date
18. After blood has infused, flush the tubing with normal saline. *Comments:*	☐	☐	☐	
19. Dispose of bag, tubing, and gloves appropriately. Wash hands. *Comments:*	☐	☐	☐	
20. Document the procedure. *Comments:*	☐	☐	☐	

_____   _____

Faculty Signature   Date

Checklist for Procedure 35-1 Inserting and Maintaining a Nasogastric Tube

Name _____ Date _____

School _____

Instructor _____

Course _____

Procedure 35-1 Inserting and Maintaining a Nasogastric Tube	Able to Perform	Able to Perform with Assistance	Unable to Perform	Initials and Date
Assessment				
1. Assess client's consciousness level. *Comments:*	☐	☐	☐	
2. Check the client's chart for any history of nostril surgery or unusual nostril bleeding. *Comments:*	☐	☐	☐	
3. Use a penlight to assess nostrils for a deviated septum. *Comments:*	☐	☐	☐	
4. Ask the client to breathe, occluding one nostril at a time. *Comments:*	☐	☐	☐	
Planning/Expected Outcomes				
1. Client's nutritional status will improve. *Comments:*	☐	☐	☐	
2. Client's nutritional needs will be met. *Comments:*	☐	☐	☐	
3. Client will maintain a patent airway. *Comments:*	☐	☐	☐	
4. Client will not have diarrhea due to nasogastric (NG) feeding. *Comments:*	☐	☐	☐	
5. Mouth mucous membranes will remain moist and intact. *Comments:*	☐	☐	☐	
6. Client will maintain a normal fluid volume. *Comments:*	☐	☐	☐	

continued on the following page

continued from the previous page

Procedure 35-1	Able to Perform	Able to Perform with Assistance	Unable to Perform	Initials and Date
7. Client's comfort level will increase. *Comments:*	☐	☐	☐	
8. Skin around the tube will remain intact. *Comments:*	☐	☐	☐	

Implementation

Procedure 35-1	Able to Perform	Able to Perform with Assistance	Unable to Perform	Initials and Date
1. Review client's medical history. *Comments:*	☐	☐	☐	
2. Explain the procedure and develop a hand signal. *Comments:*	☐	☐	☐	
3. Prepare the equipment. *Comments:*	☐	☐	☐	
4. Prepare the environment; place the bed in a high-Fowler's position. Cover the client's chest with a towel. *Comments:*	☐	☐	☐	
5. Wash hands and apply gloves. *Comments:*	☐	☐	☐	
6. Assess the client's nostrils. Have the client blow nose, one nostril at a time. *Comments:*	☐	☐	☐	
7. Measure the NG tube against the client. Mark this distance with a piece of tape. *Comments:*	☐	☐	☐	
8. Lubricate first 4 inches of the tube with water-soluble lubricant. *Comments:*	☐	☐	☐	
9. Ask the client to slightly flex the neck backward. *Comments:*	☐	☐	☐	
10. Gently insert the tube into a naris. *Comments:*	☐	☐	☐	

Procedure 35-1	Able to Perform	Able to Perform with Assistance	Unable to Perform	Initials and Date
11. Tip the client's head forward once the tube reaches the nasopharynx. If the client continues to gag, stop a moment. *Comments:*	☐	☐	☐	
12. Advance the tube several inches at a time as the client swallows. *Comments:*	☐	☐	☐	
13. Withdraw the tube immediately if there are signs of respiratory distress. *Comments:*	☐	☐	☐	
14. Advance the tube until the taped mark is reached. *Comments:*	☐	☐	☐	
15. Split a 4-inch strip of tape lengthwise 2 inches. Secure the tube with the tape. Tape to cheek as well if desired. *Comments:*	☐	☐	☐	
16. Check the placement of the tube. • Inject 10 cc of air and auscultate. • Aspirate gastric content and measure pH. • Prepare the client for x-ray check-up, if prescribed. *Comments:*	☐	☐	☐	
17. Connect the distal end of the tube to suction, draining bag, or adapter. *Comments:*	☐	☐	☐	
18. Secure the tube with a rubber band and safety pin to client's gown or bed sheet. *Comments:*	☐	☐	☐	
19. Remove gloves, dispose of used materials appropriately, and wash hands. *Comments:*	☐	☐	☐	
20. Position client comfortably with the call light within reach. *Comments:*	☐	☐	☐	
21. Document procedure. *Comments:*	☐	☐	☐	

 continued on the following page

continued from the previous page

Procedure 35-1	Able to Perform	Able to Perform with Assistance	Unable to Perform	Initials and Date
Maintaining a Nasogastric Tube 22. Wash hands and apply gloves. *Comments:*	☐	☐	☐	
23. Check tube placement (see step 16) before instilling anything per NG tube or at least every 8 hours. *Comments:*	☐	☐	☐	
24. Assess for signs that the tube has become blocked. *Comments:*	☐	☐	☐	
25. Do not irrigate or rotate a tube that has been placed during gastric or esophageal surgery. *Comments:*	☐	☐	☐	
26. Provide oral hygiene and assist client to clean nares daily. *Comments:*	☐	☐	☐	
27. Remove gloves, dispose of used materials appropriately, and wash hands. *Comments:*	☐	☐	☐	

_____   _____

Faculty Signature   Date

Checklist for Procedure 35-2   Assessing Placement of a Large-Bore Feeding Tube

Name _____ Date _____

School _____

Instructor _____

Course _____

Procedure 35-2 Assessing Placement of a Large-Bore Feeding Tube	Able to Perform	Able to Perform with Assistance	Unable to Perform	Initials and Date
Assessment				
1. Check the written order for the type and size of feeding tube to place. *Comments:*	☐	☐	☐	
2. Review the client's medical record for a history of prior tube use or displacement. *Comments:*	☐	☐	☐	
3. Assess the client for signs of inadvertent respiratory placement. *Comments:*	☐	☐	☐	
4. Assess the client for symptoms that increase the risk of tube dislocation. *Comments:*	☐	☐	☐	
Planning/Expected Outcomes				
1. The tube will remain in place and intact. *Comments:*	☐	☐	☐	
2. The tube feeding or medication will infuse into the client's gastrointestinal tract. *Comments:*	☐	☐	☐	
3. The client will not experience any respiratory distress. *Comments:*	☐	☐	☐	
4. The client will not experience any pain. *Comments:*	☐	☐	☐	
5. The client will understand the reason for checking the tube's placement. *Comments:*	☐	☐	☐	

continued on the following page

continued from the previous page

Procedure 35-2	Able to Perform	Able to Perform with Assistance	Unable to Perform	Initials and Date
Implementation				
1. Check the written order for the feeding tube. *Comments:*	☐	☐	☐	
2. Wash hands. Put on gloves. *Comments:*	☐	☐	☐	
3. Assess placement of the tube by auscultation. • Place stethoscope over left upper quadrant of the abdomen. • Quickly inject 10–20 ml air. • Assess for resistance. • Listen for sound. *Comments:*	☐	☐	☐	
4. Measure pH of gastrointestinal (GI) contents. • Aspirate 10 cc GI contents with 60-cc syringe. • If unable to aspirate, reposition client and try again. • Measure pH of GI contents with pH indicator strip. *Comments:*	☐	☐	☐	
5. Proceed with feeding and medication. Continue to monitor the client. *Comments:*	☐	☐	☐	
6. Recheck tube placement following the tube feeding. • Flush tube with 30 cc warm water after medication or tube feeding. • Wait 1 hour before testing pH. • Inject 30 cc air and auscultate for sound. • Aspirate 10 cc of GI contents and check for pH. *Comments:*	☐	☐	☐	
7. Remove gloves and wash hands. *Comments:*	☐	☐	☐	

_____   _____
Faculty Signature   Date

Checklist for Procedure 36-1   Obtaining a Wound Drainage Specimen for Culturing

Name _____ Date _____

School _____

Instructor _____

Course _____

Procedure 36-1 **Obtaining a Wound Drainage Specimen for Culturing**	Able to Perform	Able to Perform with Assistance	Unable to Perform	Initials and Date
Assessment				
1. Assess the wound and the surrounding tissues. *Comments:*	☐	☐	☐	
2. Assess the client's overall status. *Comments:*	☐	☐	☐	
Planning/Expected Outcomes				
1. The culture will be collected with a minimum of trauma to the client. *Comments:*	☐	☐	☐	
2. The culture will be representative of the wound flora. *Comments:*	☐	☐	☐	
Implementation				

1. • Wash hands and apply gloves.
    • Remove old dressing.
    • Dispose of dressing and gloves appropriately.
    • Wash hands again.
Comments:
	☐	☐	☐	

2. Open the dressing supplies aseptically and apply gloves. *Comments:*	☐	☐	☐	
3. Assess the wound's appearance. *Comments:*	☐	☐	☐	
4. Irrigate the wound with normal saline prior to collecting the culture. *Comments:*	☐	☐	☐	
5. Blot the excess saline with a sterile gauze pad. *Comments:*	☐	☐	☐	

continued on the following page

continued from the previous page

Procedure 36-1	Able to Perform	Able to Perform with Assistance	Unable to Perform	Initials and Date
6. Remove the culture swab from the tube and roll the swab over the granulation tissue. *Comments:*	☐	☐	☐	
7. • Replace the swab in the culture tube. Do not touch the swab to any surface outside of the collection tube. • Recap the tube. • Crush the medium located in the bottom or cap of the tube. *Comments:*	☐	☐	☐	
8. Remove gloves, wash hands, and apply sterile gloves. Dress the wound. *Comments:*	☐	☐	☐	
9. Label and transport the specimen to the laboratory. *Comments:*	☐	☐	☐	
10. Remove gloves and wash hands. *Comments:*	☐	☐	☐	
11. Document all assessment findings and actions taken. *Comments:*	☐	☐	☐	

_____   _____

Faculty Signature   Date

Checklist for Procedure 36-2   Irrigating a Wound

Name _____ Date _____

School _____

Instructor _____

Course _____

Procedure 36-2 **Irrigating a Wound**	Able to Perform	Able to Perform with Assistance	Unable to Perform	Initials and Date
Assessment				
1. Assess the current dressing. *Comments:*	☐	☐	☐	
2. Assess the client. *Comments:*	☐	☐	☐	
3. Assess client concerns regarding this wound and the irrigation. *Comments:*	☐	☐	☐	
4. Assess the client's environment. *Comments:*	☐	☐	☐	
Planning/Expected Outcomes				
1. The wound will be free of exudate, drainage, and debris. *Comments:*	☐	☐	☐	
2. The wound will be free of signs and symptoms of infection. *Comments:*	☐	☐	☐	
3. The procedure will be performed with a minimum of trauma to the client. *Comments:*	☐	☐	☐	
Implementation				
1. Confirm the written order for wound irrigation. *Comments:*	☐	☐	☐	
2. Assess the client's pain level and medicate if needed. *Comments:*	☐	☐	☐	
3. Explain the procedure to the client. *Comments:*	☐	☐	☐	

                    continued on the following page

continued from the previous page

Procedure 36-2	Able to Perform	Able to Perform with Assistance	Unable to Perform	Initials and Date
4. Assist the client onto a waterproof pad in a position that will allow the irrigant to flow from the clean to dirty areas of the wound. *Comments:*	☐	☐	☐	
5. Wash hands and apply gloves. Remove and discard the old dressing. *Comments:*	☐	☐	☐	
6. Assess the wound's appearance. *Comments:*	☐	☐	☐	
7. Remove and discard the gloves, and wash hands. *Comments:*	☐	☐	☐	
8. Prepare the sterile irrigation tray and dressing supplies. *Comments:*	☐	☐	☐	
9. Apply sterile gloves (and goggles if needed). *Comments:*	☐	☐	☐	
10. Pour sterile, room-temperature irrigation solution into a sterile container. *Comments:*	☐	☐	☐	
11. Position the sterile basin so the irrigant will flow into the basin. *Comments:*	☐	☐	☐	
12. Fill the syringe with irrigant and gently flush the wound. Repeat until clear or the ordered amount of fluid has been used. *Comments:*	☐	☐	☐	
13. Dry the edges of the wound with sterile gauze. *Comments:*	☐	☐	☐	
14. Assess the wound's appearance and drainage. *Comments:*	☐	☐	☐	

Procedure 36-2	Able to Perform	Able to Perform with Assistance	Unable to Perform	Initials and Date
15. Apply a sterile dressing. Remove gloves and dispose of properly. Wash hands. *Comments:*	☐	☐	☐	
16. Document all assessment findings and actions taken. *Comments:*	☐	☐	☐	

Faculty Signature

Date

Checklist for Procedure 36-3 Applying a Dry Dressing

Name _____ Date _____

School _____

Instructor _____

Course _____

Procedure 36-3 Applying a Dry Dressing	Able to Perform	Able to Perform with Assistance	Unable to Perform	Initials and Date
Assessment				
1. Assess the client's comfort level. *Comments:*	☐	☐	☐	
2. Assess the external appearance of the initial and subsequent dressings. *Comments:*	☐	☐	☐	
3. Assess the appearance of the wound and drains once the dressing is removed. *Comments:*	☐	☐	☐	
4. Assess the client's understanding about the care of the surgical site. *Comments:*	☐	☐	☐	
Planning/Expected Outcomes				
1. The site will be inspected. *Comments:*	☐	☐	☐	
2. The initial dressing will be reinforced until changed by the qualified practitioner. *Comments:*	☐	☐	☐	
3. The site will have the appropriate dressing applied. *Comments:*	☐	☐	☐	
4. The client/family will demonstrate the ability to perform the wound care and dressing change. *Comments:*	☐	☐	☐	

continued on the following page

continued from the previous page

Procedure 36-3	Able to Perform	Able to Perform with Assistance	Unable to Perform	Initials and Date
Implementation				
1. Gather supplies. *Comments:*	☐	☐	☐	
2. Provide privacy. *Comments:*	☐	☐	☐	
3. Explain procedure to client. *Comments:*	☐	☐	☐	
4. Wash hands. *Comments:*	☐	☐	☐	
5. Apply clean exam gloves. *Comments:*	☐	☐	☐	
6. Remove dressing and place in appropriate receptacle. *Comments:*	☐	☐	☐	
7. Observe the undressed wound. *Comments:*	☐	☐	☐	
8. Cleanse around the incision with a warm, wet washcloth. • Cleanse the suture line with prescribed solution. • Used applicators should not be reintroduced into the sterile solution. *Comments:*	☐	☐	☐	
9. Remove used exam gloves. *Comments:*	☐	☐	☐	
10. Wash hands. *Comments:*	☐	☐	☐	
11. Set up supplies. *Comments:*	☐	☐	☐	
12. Apply a new pair of clean exam gloves. *Comments:*	☐	☐	☐	

Procedure 36-3	Able to Perform	Able to Perform with Assistance	Unable to Perform	Initials and Date
13. Grasping just the edges, apply a new gauze dressing. Tape lightly or apply tubular mesh. *Comments:*	☐	☐	☐	
14. Mark initials, date, and time on the dressing to validate that the dressing has been changed. *Comments:*	☐	☐	☐	
15. Remove gloves and wash hands. *Comments:*	☐	☐	☐	
16. Conduct client/family education about the dressing. *Comments:*	☐	☐	☐	

_____   _____

Faculty Signature   Date

Checklist for Procedure 36-4   Applying a Wet to Damp Dressing
(Wet to Dry to Moist Dressing)

Name _____ Date _____

School _____

Instructor _____

Course _____

Procedure 36-4 Applying a Wet to Damp Dressing (Wet to Dry to Moist Dressing)	Able to Perform	Able to Perform with Assistance	Unable to Perform	Initials and Date
Assessment				
1. Assess the client's comfort level. *Comments:*	☐	☐	☐	
2. Assess the external appearance of the dressing. *Comments:*	☐	☐	☐	
3. After the dressing is removed, assess the appearance of the wound and drains. *Comments:*	☐	☐	☐	
4. Assess the client's understanding of the dressing changes and wound care. *Comments:*	☐	☐	☐	
Planning/Expected Outcomes				
1. The site will be inspected. *Comments:*	☐	☐	☐	
2. The site will have the appropriate dressing applied. *Comments:*	☐	☐	☐	
3. The client/family will demonstrate understanding and ability to perform the dressing change and wound care. *Comments:*	☐	☐	☐	
Implementation				
1. Gather supplies. *Comments:*	☐	☐	☐	
2. Provide privacy; draw curtains; close door. *Comments:*	☐	☐	☐	

    continued on the following page

continued from the previous page

Procedure 36-4	Able to Perform	Able to Perform with Assistance	Unable to Perform	Initials and Date
3. Explain procedure to client. *Comments:*	☐	☐	☐	
4. Wash hands. *Comments:*	☐	☐	☐	
5. Apply clean gloves and other needed protective clothing. *Comments:*	☐	☐	☐	
6. Assess client need for pain medication. *Comments:*	☐	☐	☐	
7. Inform client that the dressing is going to be removed. *Comments:*	☐	☐	☐	
8. Remove wet to damp dressing and dispose of appropriately. Note the makeup of the old dressing. *Comments:*	☐	☐	☐	
9. Observe the undressed wound. *Comments:*	☐	☐	☐	
10. Cleanse the skin around the incision, if necessary. *Comments:*	☐	☐	☐	
11. Remove used exam gloves. *Comments:*	☐	☐	☐	
12. Wash hands. *Comments:*	☐	☐	☐	
13. Set up supplies in a sterile field. *Comments:*	☐	☐	☐	
14. Apply sterile gloves. *Comments:*	☐	☐	☐	

Procedure 36-4	Able to Perform	Able to Perform with Assistance	Unable to Perform	Initials and Date
15. Place packing material in the bowl with the ordered solution. • Wring gauze or packing until damp. • Gently place wet gauze over the area. *Comments:*	☐	☐	☐	
16. Apply dry external dressing. • Secure dressing with tape, Montgomery straps, or tubular mesh. *Comments:*	☐	☐	☐	
17. Remove gloves and wash hands. *Comments:*	☐	☐	☐	
18. Mark the dressing with the date, time, and initials. *Comments:*	☐	☐	☐	
19. Conduct client/family education about the dressing. *Comments:*	☐	☐	☐	

Faculty Signature   Date

Checklist for Procedure 37-1　Assisting with a Bedpan or Urinal

Name _____　Date _____

School _____

Instructor _____

Course _____

Procedure 37-1 **Assisting with a Bedpan or Urinal**	Able to Perform	Able to Perform with Assistance	Unable to Perform	Initials and Date
Assessment				
1. Gather your equipment. *Comments:*	☐	☐	☐	
2. Assess how much the client can assist with the procedure. *Comments:*	☐	☐	☐	
3. Assess whether the client is confused, combative, or immobile. *Comments:*	☐	☐	☐	
4. Check for casts, braces, or dressings. *Comments:*	☐	☐	☐	
5. Check for privacy and unexpected interruptions. *Comments:*	☐	☐	☐	
Planning/Expected Outcomes				
1. Client will be able to void and defecate when necessary. *Comments:*	☐	☐	☐	
2. Client will have as much privacy and comfort as allowable. *Comments:*	☐	☐	☐	
3. Intake and output will be accurately measured as needed. *Comments:*	☐	☐	☐	
4. The urinal or bedpan will be placed without skin damage. *Comments:*	☐	☐	☐	
5. The bedpan will be removed and emptied without spillage. *Comments:*	☐	☐	☐	

　　　　continued on the following page

continued from the previous page

Procedure 37-1	Able to Perform	Able to Perform with Assistance	Unable to Perform	Initials and Date
Implementation				
Positioning a Bedpan				
1. Close curtain or door. *Comments:*	☐	☐	☐	
2. Wash hands; apply gloves. *Comments:*	☐	☐	☐	
3. Lower head of bed so client is in supine position. *Comments:*	☐	☐	☐	
4. Elevate bed. *Comments:*	☐	☐	☐	
5. Assist client to side-lying position. *Comments:*	☐	☐	☐	
6. Warm and powder bedpan, if necessary. *Comments:*	☐	☐	☐	
7. Place bedpan under buttocks. *Comments:*	☐	☐	☐	
8. Help the client roll onto the back with the bedpan in place. *Comments:*	☐	☐	☐	
9. Alternate: Help the client raise the hips and slide the pan in place. Alternate: Use a fracture pan instead of a bedpan. *Comments:*	☐	☐	☐	
10. Check placement of bedpan. *Comments:*	☐	☐	☐	
11. If indicated, elevate head of bed to 45° angle. *Comments:*	☐	☐	☐	
12. Place call light within reach; provide for client safety and privacy. *Comments:*	☐	☐	☐	

Procedure 37-1	Able to Perform	Able to Perform with Assistance	Unable to Perform	Initials and Date
13. Remove gloves; wash hands. *Comments:*	☐	☐	☐	
Positioning a Urinal 14. Close curtain or door. Wash hands; apply gloves. *Comments:*	☐	☐	☐	
15. Lift the covers. Allow client to place urinal or place it yourself. *Comments:*	☐	☐	☐	
16. Remove gloves; wash hands. *Comments:*	☐	☐	☐	
Removing a Bedpan 17. Wash hands; apply gloves. *Comments:*	☐	☐	☐	
18. Gather toilet paper and washing supplies. *Comments:*	☐	☐	☐	
19. Lower head of bed to supine position. *Comments:*	☐	☐	☐	
20. Roll client to side and remove the pan. *Comments:*	☐	☐	☐	
21. Assist with cleaning or wiping. *Comments:*	☐	☐	☐	
22. Measure output. Empty, clean, and store bedpan in proper place. *Comments:*	☐	☐	☐	
23. Remove soiled gloves. Wash hands. *Comments:*	☐	☐	☐	
24. Allow client to wash hands. *Comments:*	☐	☐	☐	

 continued on the following page

continued from the previous page

Procedure 37-1	Able to Perform	Able to Perform with Assistance	Unable to Perform	Initials and Date
25. Place call light within reach; put side rails up; lower bed. *Comments:*	☐	☐	☐	
26. Wash hands. *Comments:*	☐	☐	☐	
Removing a Urinal 27. Wash hands and apply gloves. Remove the urinal. *Comments:*	☐	☐	☐	
28. Measure urine output. Empty and rinse the urinal. Place it in the client's reach. *Comments:*	☐	☐	☐	
29. Remove soiled gloves. Wash hands. *Comments:*	☐	☐	☐	
30. Allow client to wash hands. *Comments:*	☐	☐	☐	
31. Place call light within reach; put side rails up. *Comments:*	☐	☐	☐	
32. Wash hands. *Comments:*	☐	☐	☐	

Faculty Signature

Date

Checklist for Procedure 37-2   Applying a Condom Catheter

Name _____ Date _____

School _____

Instructor _____

Course _____

Procedure 37-2 **Applying a Condom Catheter**	Able to Perform	Able to Perform with Assistance	Unable to Perform	Initials and Date
Assessment				
1. Assess skin integrity around the penis and perineal area. *Comments:*	☐	☐	☐	
2. Assess the client for ability to cooperate. *Comments:*	☐	☐	☐	
3. Assess the amount and pattern of urinary incontinence. *Comments:*	☐	☐	☐	
Planning/Expected Outcomes				
1. The client will have a condom catheter in place. *Comments:*	☐	☐	☐	
2. The client will have no skin irritation. *Comments:*	☐	☐	☐	
3. The client will understand and cooperate with placement and retention of the condom catheter. *Comments:*	☐	☐	☐	
Implementation				
1. Wash hands. *Comments:*	☐	☐	☐	
2. Provide privacy. *Comments:*	☐	☐	☐	
3. Position the client comfortably. Raise the bed to a comfortable height for the nurse. *Comments:*	☐	☐	☐	

   continued on the following page

continued from the previous page

Procedure 37-2	Able to Perform	Able to Perform with Assistance	Unable to Perform	Initials and Date
4. Apply gloves. *Comments:*	☐	☐	☐	
5. Fold the client's gown across the abdomen and pull the sheet up over the client's legs. *Comments:*	☐	☐	☐	
6. Assess the client's penis. *Comments:*	☐	☐	☐	
7. Clean the client's penis with warm soapy water. *Comments:*	☐	☐	☐	
8. Return the client's foreskin to its normal position. *Comments:*	☐	☐	☐	
9. Shave any excess hair around the base of the penis. *Comments:*	☐	☐	☐	
10. Rinse and dry the area. *Comments:*	☐	☐	☐	
11. If a condom kit is used, apply skin preparation solution to the shaft of the penis. *Comments:*	☐	☐	☐	
12. Apply the double-sided adhesive strip around the base of the client's penis in a spiral fashion. *Comments:*	☐	☐	☐	
13. Position the rolled condom at the distal portion of the penis and unroll it, covering the penis and the double-sided strip of adhesive. *Comments:*	☐	☐	☐	
14. Gently press the condom to the adhesive strip. *Comments:*	☐	☐	☐	

Procedure 37-2	Able to Perform	Able to Perform with Assistance	Unable to Perform	Initials and Date
15. Attach the drainage bag tubing to the catheter tubing. Secure the drainage bag. *Comments:*	☐	☐	☐	
16. Determine that the condom and tubing are not twisted. *Comments:*	☐	☐	☐	
17. Cover the client. *Comments:*	☐	☐	☐	
18. Dispose of the used equipment appropriately and wash hands. *Comments:*	☐	☐	☐	
19. Return the client's bed to the lowest position and reposition client comfortably. *Comments:*	☐	☐	☐	
20. Empty the bag, measure the urinary output, and record every 4 hours. *Comments:*	☐	☐	☐	
21. Remove the condom once a day to clean the area and assess the skin. *Comments:*	☐	☐	☐	

_____   _____
Faculty Signature   Date

Checklist for Procedure 37-3   Inserting an Indwelling Catheter: Male

Name _____ Date _____

School _____

Instructor _____

Course _____

Procedure 37-3 **Inserting an Indwelling Catheter: Male**	Able to Perform	Able to Perform with Assistance	Unable to Perform	Initials and Date
Assessment				
1. Assess the need for catheterization and the type of catheterization ordered. *Comments:*	☐	☐	☐	
2. Assess the need for peritoneal care prior to catheterization. *Comments:*	☐	☐	☐	
3. Assess the urinary meatus. Ask the client for any history of difficulty with prior catheterizations. *Comments:*	☐	☐	☐	
4. Assess the client's ability to assist with the procedure. *Comments:*	☐	☐	☐	
5. Assess the light. *Comments:*	☐	☐	☐	
6. Assess for an allergy to povidone-iodine. *Comments:*	☐	☐	☐	
7. Observe for indications of distress or embarrassment. *Comments:*	☐	☐	☐	
Planning/Expected Outcomes				
1. The catheter will be inserted without trauma to the client. *Comments:*	☐	☐	☐	
2. The client's bladder will be emptied without complication. *Comments:*	☐	☐	☐	
3. The nurse will maintain the sterility of the catheter during insertion. *Comments:*	☐	☐	☐	

                              continued on the following page

continued from the previous page

Procedure 37-3	Able to Perform	Able to Perform with Assistance	Unable to Perform	Initials and Date
Implementation				
1. Gather the equipment needed. *Comments:*	☐	☐	☐	
2. Provide for privacy and explain procedure to client. *Comments:*	☐	☐	☐	
3. Set the bed to a comfortable height to work, and raise the opposite side rail. *Comments:*	☐	☐	☐	
4. Assist the client to a supine position with legs slightly spread. *Comments:*	☐	☐	☐	
5. Drape the client's abdomen and thighs if needed. *Comments:*	☐	☐	☐	
6. Ensure adequate lighting of the penis and perineal area. *Comments:*	☐	☐	☐	
7. Wash hands, apply disposable gloves, and wash perineal area. *Comments:*	☐	☐	☐	
8. Remove gloves and wash hands. *Comments:*	☐	☐	☐	
9. Open the catheterization kit. Use the wrapper to establish a sterile field. *Comments:*	☐	☐	☐	
10. Add the catheter or any other items needed using sterile technique. *Comments:*	☐	☐	☐	
11. Apply sterile gloves. *Comments:*	☐	☐	☐	

Procedure 37-3	Able to Perform	Able to Perform with Assistance	Unable to Perform	Initials and Date
12. Place the fenestrated drape over the client's perineal area with the penis extending through the opening. *Comments:*	☐	☐	☐	
13. If inserting a retention catheter, attach the syringe filled with sterile water to the Luer-Lok tail of the catheter. Inflate and deflate the retention balloon. Detach the water-filled syringe. *Comments:*	☐	☐	☐	
14. Attach the catheter to the urine drainage bag. *Comments:*	☐	☐	☐	
15. Coat the distal portion of the catheter with water-soluble, sterile lubricant. *Comments:*	☐	☐	☐	
16. With one hand, gently grasp the penis and retract the foreskin (if present). With your other hand, cleanse the glans penis with antimicrobial cleanser. *Comments:*	☐	☐	☐	
17. Hold the penis perpendicular to the body and gently pull up. *Comments:*	☐	☐	☐	
18. Inject 10 ml sterile, water-soluble lubricant into the urethra. *Comments:*	☐	☐	☐	
19. Steadily insert the catheter about 8 inches, until urine is noted. *Comments:*	☐	☐	☐	
20. If the catheter will be removed right away, insert the catheter another inch, place the penis in a comfortable position and hold the catheter in place as the bladder drains into a sterile receptacle. *Comments:*	☐	☐	☐	

continued on the following page

continued from the previous page

Procedure 37-3	Able to Perform	Able to Perform with Assistance	Unable to Perform	Initials and Date
21. If the catheter will be indwelling with a retention balloon, continue inserting until the hub of the catheter is met. *Comments:*	☐	☐	☐	
22. Reattach the water-filled syringe to the inflation port. *Comments:*	☐	☐	☐	
23. Inflate the retention balloon. *Comments:*	☐	☐	☐	
24. If the client experiences pain during balloon inflation, deflate the balloon and insert the catheter farther into the bladder. If the pain continues with balloon inflation, remove the catheter and notify the client's qualified practitioner. *Comments:*	☐	☐	☐	
25. Once the balloon has been inflated, gently pull the catheter until the retention balloon is resting against the bladder neck. *Comments:*	☐	☐	☐	
26. Secure the catheter to either the client's thigh or abdomen. *Comments:*	☐	☐	☐	
27. Place the drainage bag below the level of the bladder. Secure the drainage tubing to prevent pulling. *Comments:*	☐	☐	☐	
28. Remove gloves, dispose of equipment, and wash hands. *Comments:*	☐	☐	☐	
29. Help client adjust position. Lower the bed. *Comments:*	☐	☐	☐	
30. Assess and document properties of the client's urine. *Comments:*	☐	☐	☐	

_____   _____

Faculty Signature   Date

Checklist for Procedure 37-4   Inserting an Indwelling Catheter: Female

Name _____ Date _____

School _____

Instructor _____

Course _____

Procedure 37-4 Inserting an Indwelling Catheter: Female	Able to Perform	Able to Perform with Assistance	Unable to Perform	Initials and Date
Assessment				
1. Assess the need for catheterization and the type of catheterization ordered. *Comments:*	☐	☐	☐	
2. Assess for the need for peritoneal care prior to catheterization. *Comments:*	☐	☐	☐	
3. Assess the urinary meatus. Ask the client for any history of difficulty with prior catheterizations. *Comments:*	☐	☐	☐	
4. Assess the client's ability to assist with the procedure. *Comments:*	☐	☐	☐	
5. Assess the light. *Comments:*	☐	☐	☐	
6. Assess for an allergy to povidone-iodine. *Comments:*	☐	☐	☐	
7. Observe for indications of distress or embarrassment. *Comments:*	☐	☐	☐	
Planning/Expected Outcomes				
1. The catheter will be inserted without trauma to the client. *Comments:*	☐	☐	☐	
2. The client's bladder will be emptied without complication. *Comments:*	☐	☐	☐	
3. The nurse will maintain the sterility of the catheter during insertion. *Comments:*	☐	☐	☐	

   continued on the following page

continued from the previous page

Procedure 37-4	Able to Perform	Able to Perform with Assistance	Unable to Perform	Initials and Date
Implementation				
1. Gather the equipment needed. *Comments:*	☐	☐	☐	
2. Provide for privacy and explain procedure to client. *Comments:*	☐	☐	☐	
3. Set the bed to a comfortable height to work, and raise the opposite side rail. *Comments:*	☐	☐	☐	
4. Assist the client to a supine position with legs spread or to a side-lying position with upper leg flexed. *Comments:*	☐	☐	☐	
5. Drape the client's abdomen and thighs for warmth if needed. *Comments:*	☐	☐	☐	
6. Ensure adequate lighting of the perineal area. *Comments:*	☐	☐	☐	
7. Wash hands; apply disposable gloves. *Comments:*	☐	☐	☐	
8. Wash perineal area. *Comments:*	☐	☐	☐	
9. Remove gloves and wash hands. *Comments:*	☐	☐	☐	
10. Open the catheterization kit. Use the wrapper to establish a sterile field. *Comments:*	☐	☐	☐	
11. Add the catheter or any other items needed using sterile technique. *Comments:*	☐	☐	☐	
12. Apply sterile gloves. *Comments:*	☐	☐	☐	

Procedure 37-4	Able to Perform	Able to Perform with Assistance	Unable to Perform	Initials and Date
13. If inserting a retention catheter, attach the syringe filled with sterile water to the Luer-Lok tail of the catheter. Inflate and deflate the retention balloon. Detach the water-filled syringe. *Comments:*	☐	☐	☐	
14. Attach the catheter to the urine drainage bag. *Comments:*	☐	☐	☐	
15. Coat the distal portion of the catheter with water-soluble, sterile lubricant. *Comments:*	☐	☐	☐	
16. Place the fenestrated drape over the client's perineal area with the labia visible through the opening. *Comments:*	☐	☐	☐	
17. Gently spread the labia minora with your fingers and visualize the urinary meatus. *Comments:*	☐	☐	☐	
18. Holding the labia apart, use the forceps to pick up a cotton ball soaked in povidone-iodine and cleanse the periurethral mucosa using one downward stroke for each cotton ball, then dispose. *Comments:*	☐	☐	☐	
19. Steadily insert the catheter into the meatus until urine is noted. *Comments:*	☐	☐	☐	
20. If the catheter will be removed as soon as the client's bladder is empty, insert the catheter another inch and hold the catheter in place as the bladder drains into a sterile receptacle. *Comments:*	☐	☐	☐	
21. If the catheter will be indwelling with a retention balloon, continue inserting another 1 to 3 inches. *Comments:*	☐	☐	☐	

continued on the following page

continued from the previous page

Procedure 37-4	Able to Perform	Able to Perform with Assistance	Unable to Perform	Initials and Date
22. Reattach the water-filled syringe to the inflation port. *Comments:*	☐	☐	☐	
23. Inflate the retention balloon. *Comments:*	☐	☐	☐	
24. If the client experiences pain during balloon inflation, deflate the balloon and insert the catheter farther into the bladder. If the pain continues with balloon inflation, remove the catheter and notify the client's qualified practitioner. *Comments:*	☐	☐	☐	
25. Once the balloon has been inflated, gently pull the catheter until the retention balloon is resting against the bladder neck. *Comments:*	☐	☐	☐	
26. Tape the catheter to the abdomen or thigh with enough slack so it will not pull on the bladder. *Comments:*	☐	☐	☐	
27. Place the drainage bag below the level of the bladder. *Comments:*	☐	☐	☐	
28. Remove gloves, dispose of equipment, and wash hands. *Comments:*	☐	☐	☐	
29. Help client adjust position. Lower the bed. *Comments:*	☐	☐	☐	
30. Wash hands. *Comments:*	☐	☐	☐	
31. Assess and document the urine's properties. *Comments:*	☐	☐	☐	

_____   _____
Faculty Signature   Date

Checklist for Procedure 37-5   Irrigating a Urinary Catheter

Name _____ Date _____

School _____

Instructor _____

Course _____

Procedure 37-5 **Irrigating a Urinary Catheter**	Able to Perform	Able to Perform with Assistance	Unable to Perform	Initials and Date
Assessment				
1. Assess the written order for type and purpose of the irrigation. *Comments:*	☐	☐	☐	
2. Assess the condition of the client. *Comments:*	☐	☐	☐	
3. Assess for current pain or bladder spasms. *Comments:*	☐	☐	☐	
4. Assess client's knowledge about the procedure. *Comments:*	☐	☐	☐	
5. If this is a repeat of the procedure, read the charting by previous nurses. *Comments:*	☐	☐	☐	
Planning/Expected Outcomes				
1. Urinary catheter will be patent. *Comments:*	☐	☐	☐	
2. Sediment/blood clots will be passed through the catheter. *Comments:*	☐	☐	☐	
3. Bladder will be free of sources of local irritation. *Comments:*	☐	☐	☐	
4. Urinary pH will be assisted to a more acidic state. *Comments:*	☐	☐	☐	

continued on the following page

continued from the previous page

Procedure 37-5	Able to Perform	Able to Perform with Assistance	Unable to Perform	Initials and Date
Implementation				
1. Verify the need for bladder or catheter irrigation. *Comments:*	☐	☐	☐	
2. For prn irrigation, palpate for full bladder and check current output against previous totals. *Comments:*	☐	☐	☐	
3. Verify written orders for type of irrigation and irrigant, as well as amount. *Comments:*	☐	☐	☐	
4. If repeat procedure, read previous documentation in the record. *Comments:*	☐	☐	☐	
5. Assemble all supplies. *Comments:*	☐	☐	☐	
6. Premedicate client if ordered or needed. *Comments:*	☐	☐	☐	
7. Provide teaching to the client as needed. *Comments:*	☐	☐	☐	
8. Assist the client to a dorsal recumbent position. *Comments:*	☐	☐	☐	
9. Wash your hands. *Comments:*	☐	☐	☐	
10. Provide for client privacy. *Comments:*	☐	☐	☐	
11. Empty the collection bag of urine. *Comments:*	☐	☐	☐	
12. Expose the retention catheter, and place the water-resistant drape underneath it. *Comments:*	☐	☐	☐	

Procedure 37-5	Able to Perform	Able to Perform with Assistance	Unable to Perform	Initials and Date
13. Open the sterile syringe and container. Stand sterile container with syringe up and add 100–200 cc sterile diluent. *Comments:*	☐	☐	☐	
14. Open the antiseptic swab package, exposing the swab sticks. *Comments:*	☐	☐	☐	
15. Open the sterile cover for drainage tube. *Comments:*	☐	☐	☐	
16. Apply the sterile gloves. *Comments:*	☐	☐	☐	
17. Disinfect the connection between the catheter and the drainage tubing. *Comments:*	☐	☐	☐	
18. Loosen the ends of the connection. *Comments:*	☐	☐	☐	
19. Grasp the catheter and tubing 1 to 2 inches from their ends, with the catheter in the nondominant hand. *Comments:*	☐	☐	☐	
20. Pinch the catheter closed; use the thumb and first finger to hold the sterile cap for the drainage tube. *Comments:*	☐	☐	☐	
21. Separate the catheter and tube, covering the tube tightly with the sterile cap. *Comments:*	☐	☐	☐	
22. Fill the syringe with irrigant. Insert the tip of the syringe into the catheter and instill the solution into the catheter. *Comments:*	☐	☐	☐	
23. Clamp catheter if ordered; if not, drain or aspirate irrigant. *Comments:*	☐	☐	☐	

continued on the following page

continued from the previous page

Procedure 37-5	Able to Perform	Able to Perform with Assistance	Unable to Perform	Initials and Date
24. If irrigation is to clear solid material, repeat irrigation until return is clear. *Comments:*	☐	☐	☐	
25. Reconnect system and remove sterile gloves. Wash your hands. *Comments:*	☐	☐	☐	
26. Chart type of returns and total amount of irrigation fluid used. *Comments:*	☐	☐	☐	
27. Monitor client's condition. *Comments:*	☐	☐	☐	
28. Wash hands. *Comments:*	☐	☐	☐	

_____   _____
Faculty Signature   Date

Checklist for Procedure 37-6   Irrigating the Bladder Using a Closed-System Catheter

Name _____ Date _____

School _____

Instructor _____

Course _____

Procedure 37-6 **Irrigating the Bladder Using a Closed-System Catheter**	Able to Perform	Able to Perform with Assistance	Unable to Perform	Initials and Date
Assessment				
1. Assess for bladder distention or complaints of fullness. *Comments:*	☐	☐	☐	
2. Assess the drainage system for equal or larger amounts of drainage versus infused irrigant. *Comments:*	☐	☐	☐	
3. Assess the bladder drainage noting any clots or debris present. *Comments:*	☐	☐	☐	
Planning/Expected Outcomes				
1. The client will not exhibit symptoms of infection. *Comments:*	☐	☐	☐	
2. The client will not experience pain or discomfort. *Comments:*	☐	☐	☐	
3. The catheter will remain patent, and the bladder will not be distended. *Comments:*	☐	☐	☐	
Implementation				
Intermittent Bladder Irrigation Using a Standard Retention Catheter and a Y Adapter				
1. Close privacy curtain or door. *Comments:*	☐	☐	☐	
2. Wash hands. *Comments:*	☐	☐	☐	
3. Hang the prescribed irrigation solution from an IV pole. *Comments:*	☐	☐	☐	

continued on the following page

continued from the previous page

Procedure 37-6	Able to Perform	Able to Perform with Assistance	Unable to Perform	Initials and Date
4. Insert the clamped irrigation tubing into the irrigant and prime the tubing with fluid. *Comments:*	☐	☐	☐	
5. Prepare sterile antiseptic swabs and sterile Y connector. *Comments:*	☐	☐	☐	
6. Apply sterile gloves. *Comments:*	☐	☐	☐	
7. Clamp the urinary catheter. *Comments:*	☐	☐	☐	
8. Unhook the drainage bag from the retention catheter. *Comments:*	☐	☐	☐	
9. Cleanse both the drainage tubing and the drainage port with antiseptic swabs. *Comments:*	☐	☐	☐	
10. Connect the Y connector to the drainage port of the retention catheter. *Comments:*	☐	☐	☐	
11. Connect the Y adapter to the drainage tubing and bag. *Comments:*	☐	☐	☐	
12. Attach the third port of the Y adapter to the irrigant tubing. *Comments:*	☐	☐	☐	
13. Unclamp the catheter and reestablish urine drainage. *Comments:*	☐	☐	☐	
14. To irrigate the catheter and bladder, clamp the drainage tubing. *Comments:*	☐	☐	☐	
15. Infuse the prescribed amount of irrigant. *Comments:*	☐	☐	☐	

Procedure 37-6	Able to Perform	Able to Perform with Assistance	Unable to Perform	Initials and Date
16. Clamp the irrigant tubing. *Comments:*	☐	☐	☐	
17. If the irrigant is to remain in the bladder for a measured length of time, wait the prescribed length of time. *Comments:*	☐	☐	☐	
18. Unclamp the drainage tubing and monitor the drainage. *Comments:*	☐	☐	☐	
Closed Bladder Irrigation Using a Three-Way Catheter 19. Close privacy curtain or door. *Comments:*	☐	☐	☐	
20. Wash hands. *Comments:*	☐	☐	☐	
21. Explain the procedure to the client. *Comments:*	☐	☐	☐	
22. Hang the prescribed irrigation solution from an IV pole. *Comments:*	☐	☐	☐	
23. Insert the clamped irrigation tubing into the bottle of irrigant and prime the tubing. *Comments:*	☐	☐	☐	
24. Prepare sterile antiseptic swabs and other sterile equipment. *Comments:*	☐	☐	☐	
25. Apply sterile gloves. *Comments:*	☐	☐	☐	
26. Clamp the urinary catheter. *Comments:*	☐	☐	☐	
27. Remove the cap from the irrigation port of the three-way catheter. *Comments:*	☐	☐	☐	

　　　continued on the following page

continued from the previous page

Procedure 37-6	Able to Perform	Able to Perform with Assistance	Unable to Perform	Initials and Date
28. Cleanse the irrigation port with the sterile antiseptic swabs. *Comments:*	☐	☐	☐	
29. Attach the irrigation tubing to the irrigation port of the three-way catheter. *Comments:*	☐	☐	☐	
30. Remove the clamp from the catheter and observe for urine drainage. *Comments:*	☐	☐	☐	
31. If intermittent irrigation has been ordered, infuse the prescribed amount of irrigant. *Comments:*	☐	☐	☐	
32. Clamp the irrigant tubing. *Comments:*	☐	☐	☐	
33. If the irrigant is to remain in the bladder for a measured time, clamp the drainage tube prior to infusing the irrigant and wait the prescribed length of time. *Comments:*	☐	☐	☐	
34. Monitor the drainage as it flows into the drainage bag. *Comments:*	☐	☐	☐	
35. If continuous bladder irrigation has been ordered, adjust the clamp on the irrigation tubing so the prescribed rate of irrigant flows. *Comments:*	☐	☐	☐	
36. Monitor the drainage as it flows back into the drainage bag. *Comments:*	☐	☐	☐	
37. Tape the catheter securely to the thigh. *Comments:*	☐	☐	☐	
38. Wash hands. *Comments:*	☐	☐	☐	

Faculty Signature   Date

Checklist for Procedure 37-7　　Administering an Enema

Name _____ Date _____

School _____

Instructor _____

Course _____

Procedure 37-7 Administering an Enema	Able to Perform	Able to Perform with Assistance	Unable to Perform	Initials and Date
Assessment				
1. Identify the type of enema and rationale of the ordered enema. *Comments:*	☐	☐	☐	
2. Assess the physical condition of the client. *Comments:*	☐	☐	☐	
3. Assess the client's mental state. *Comments:*	☐	☐	☐	
Planning/Expected Outcomes				
1. The client's rectum will be free of feces and flatus. *Comments:*	☐	☐	☐	
2. The client will experience a minimum of trauma and embarrassment. *Comments:*	☐	☐	☐	
Implementation				
Large Volume, Cleansing Enema 1. Wash hands. *Comments:*	☐	☐	☐	
2. Assess client's understanding of procedure. Provide privacy. *Comments:*	☐	☐	☐	
3. Apply gloves. *Comments:*	☐	☐	☐	
4. Prepare equipment. *Comments:*	☐	☐	☐	

　　　　continued on the following page

continued from the previous page

Procedure 37-7	Able to Perform	Able to Perform with Assistance	Unable to Perform	Initials and Date
5. Place absorbent pad on bed under client. Assist client into left lateral position. *Comments:*	☐	☐	☐	
6. Heat solution to desired temperature. *Comments:*	☐	☐	☐	
7. Pour solution into the bag or bucket. Open clamp and prime tubing. *Comments:*	☐	☐	☐	
8. Lubricate 5 cm of the rectal tube unless the tube is prelubricated. *Comments:*	☐	☐	☐	
9. Hold the enema container level with the rectum. Have the client take a deep breath. Simultaneously insert rectal tube 7–10 cm into rectum. *Comments:*	☐	☐	☐	
10. Raise the container to the appropriate height (12 to 18 inches) and open clamp. *Comments:*	☐	☐	☐	
11. Slowly administer the fluid. *Comments:*	☐	☐	☐	
12. When solution has been administered or the client cannot hold more fluid, clamp and remove the rectal tube, disposing of it properly. *Comments:*	☐	☐	☐	
13. Clean lubricant, solution, and any feces from the anus with toilet tissue. *Comments:*	☐	☐	☐	
14. Have the client continue to lie on the left side for the prescribed length of time. *Comments:*	☐	☐	☐	
15. When the enema has been retained the prescribed amount of time, assist client to the bedside commode, toilet, or bedpan. Instruct client not to flush the toilet. *Comments:*	☐	☐	☐	

Procedure 37-7	Able to Perform	Able to Perform with Assistance	Unable to Perform	Initials and Date
16. When the client is finished, assist to clean the perineal area. *Comments:*	☐	☐	☐	
17. Return the client to a comfortable position with a protective pad in place. *Comments:*	☐	☐	☐	
18. Observe feces. *Comments:*	☐	☐	☐	
19. Remove gloves and wash hands. *Comments:*	☐	☐	☐	
20. Document the procedure and results. *Comments:*	☐	☐	☐	
Small Volume, Prepackaged Enema 21. Wash hands. *Comments:*	☐	☐	☐	
22. Remove prepackaged enema from packaging. Warm the fluid prior to use. *Comments:*	☐	☐	☐	
23. Apply gloves. *Comments:*	☐	☐	☐	
24. Place absorbent pad under client. Assist client into left lateral position. *Comments:*	☐	☐	☐	
25. Remove the protective cap from the nozzle. Lubricate as needed. *Comments:*	☐	☐	☐	
26. Squeeze the container to remove any air and prime the nozzle. *Comments:*	☐	☐	☐	
27. Have the client take a deep breath. Insert the enema nozzle into the anus. *Comments:*	☐	☐	☐	

  continued on the following page

continued from the previous page

Procedure 37-7	Able to Perform	Able to Perform with Assistance	Unable to Perform	Initials and Date
28. Squeeze the container until all the solution is instilled. *Comments:*	☐	☐	☐	
29. Remove the nozzle from the anus and dispose of the container appropriately. *Comments:*	☐	☐	☐	
30. Clean lubricant, solution, and any feces from the anus with toilet tissue. *Comments:*	☐	☐	☐	
31. Have the client continue to lie on the left side for the prescribed length of time. *Comments:*	☐	☐	☐	
32. After the prescribed amount of time, assist client to the commode, toilet, or bedpan. Instruct client not to flush the toilet. *Comments:*	☐	☐	☐	
33. When the client is finished, assist to clean the perineal area. *Comments:*	☐	☐	☐	
34. Return the client to a comfortable position on a protective pad. *Comments:*	☐	☐	☐	
35. Observe feces. *Comments:*	☐	☐	☐	
36. Remove gloves and wash hands. *Comments:*	☐	☐	☐	
37. Document procedure and record results. *Comments:*	☐	☐	☐	
Return-Flow Enema 38. Wash hands. *Comments:*	☐	☐	☐	

Procedure 37-7	Able to Perform	Able to Perform with Assistance	Unable to Perform	Initials and Date
39. Assess if client understands procedure. *Comments:*	☐	☐	☐	
40. Apply gloves. *Comments:*	☐	☐	☐	
41. Place absorbent pad on bed under client and assist into left lateral position. *Comments:*	☐	☐	☐	
42. Heat solution to desired temperature. *Comments:*	☐	☐	☐	
43. Pour solution into the bag or bucket, open clamp, and prime tubing. Clamp tubing when primed. *Comments:*	☐	☐	☐	
44. Lubricate 5 cm of the rectal tube unless the tube is prelubricated. *Comments:*	☐	☐	☐	
45. Hold the enema container level with the rectum. Have the client take a deep breath. Simultaneously insert rectal tube into rectum. *Comments:*	☐	☐	☐	
46. Raise the solution container to the appropriate height and open clamp. *Comments:*	☐	☐	☐	
47. Slowly administer approximately 200 cc of solution. *Comments:*	☐	☐	☐	
48. Clamp the tubing and lower the enema container 12 to 18 inches below the client's rectum. Open the clamp. *Comments:*	☐	☐	☐	
49. Observe the solution container for air bubbles and fecal particles as the solution returns. *Comments:*	☐	☐	☐	

　　　　　continued on the following page

continued from the previous page

Procedure 37-7	Able to Perform	Able to Perform with Assistance	Unable to Perform	Initials and Date
50. When no further solution is returned, clamp the tubing and raise the enema container as before. Open the clamp and instill approximately 200 cc of fluid. *Comments:*	☐	☐	☐	
51. Repeat until no further flatus is seen or the institutional guidelines have been met. *Comments:*	☐	☐	☐	
52. After the final return, clamp the tubing and remove the tubing. Clean the anus with tissue. *Comments:*	☐	☐	☐	
53. If the client needs to empty his rectum, assist him to the bedpan, bathroom, or commode. Instruct client not to flush the toilet. *Comments:*	☐	☐	☐	
54. When the client is finished, assist him to clean the perineal area. *Comments:*	☐	☐	☐	
55. Return the client to a comfortable position on a protective pad. *Comments:*	☐	☐	☐	
56. Observe any expelled solution. *Comments:*	☐	☐	☐	
57. Remove gloves and wash hands. *Comments:*	☐	☐	☐	
58. Document the results of the enema. *Comments:*	☐	☐	☐	

_____   _____

Faculty Signature   Date

Checklist for Procedure 37-8   Changing a Bowel Diversion Ostomy Appliance: Pouching a Stoma

Name _____ Date _____

School _____

Instructor _____

Course _____

Procedure 37-8 Changing a Bowel Diversion Ostomy Appliance: Pouching a Stoma	Able to Perform	Able to Perform with Assistance	Unable to Perform	Initials and Date
Assessment				
1. Inspect the stoma for color and texture. *Comments:*	☐	☐	☐	
2. Inspect the condition of the skin surrounding the stoma. *Comments:*	☐	☐	☐	
3. Measure the dimensions of the stoma. *Comments:*	☐	☐	☐	
Planning/Expected Outcomes				
1. Peristomal skin integrity will remain intact. *Comments:*	☐	☐	☐	
2. Irritated or denuded peristomal skin integrity will heal. *Comments:*	☐	☐	☐	
3. Client will acknowledge the change in body image. *Comments:*	☐	☐	☐	
4. Client will express positive feelings about self. *Comments:*	☐	☐	☐	
5. Client will maintain fluid balance. *Comments:*	☐	☐	☐	
Implementation				
1. Wash hands. *Comments:*	☐	☐	☐	
2. Assemble drainable pouch and wafer. *Comments:*	☐	☐	☐	

     continued on the following page

continued from the previous page

Procedure 37-8	Able to Perform	Able to Perform with Assistance	Unable to Perform	Initials and Date
3. Apply gloves. *Comments:*	☐	☐	☐	
4. Remove current ostomy appliance after emptying pouch. *Comments:*	☐	☐	☐	
5. Dispose of appliance appropriately. *Comments:*	☐	☐	☐	
6. Wash hands. *Comments:*	☐	☐	☐	
7. Apply clean gloves. *Comments:*	☐	☐	☐	
8. Cleanse stoma and skin with warm tap water. Pat dry. *Comments:*	☐	☐	☐	
9. Measure stoma at base. *Comments:*	☐	☐	☐	
10. Place gauze pad over stoma while you are preparing the new wafer and pouch. *Comments:*	☐	☐	☐	
11. Trace pattern onto paper backing of wafer. *Comments:*	☐	☐	☐	
12. Cut wafer as traced. *Comments:*	☐	☐	☐	
13. Attach clean pouch to wafer. Make sure port is closed. *Comments:*	☐	☐	☐	
14. Remove gauze pad from orifice of stoma. *Comments:*	☐	☐	☐	
15. Remove paper backing from wafer and place on skin with stoma centered in cutout opening of wafer. *Comments:*	☐	☐	☐	

Procedure 37-8	Able to Perform	Able to Perform with Assistance	Unable to Perform	Initials and Date
16. Tape the wafer edges down with hypoallergenic tape. *Comments:*	☐	☐	☐	
17. Wash hands. *Comments:*	☐	☐	☐	

Faculty Signature _____

Date _____

Checklist for Procedure 38-1   Proper Body Mechanics and Safe Lifting

Name _____ Date _____

School _____

Instructor _____

Course _____

Procedure 38-1 **Proper Body Mechanics and Safe Lifting**	Able to Perform	Able to Perform with Assistance	Unable to Perform	Initials and Date
Assessment				
1. Assess the need and degree to which the client requires assistance. *Comments:*	☐	☐	☐	
2. Identify the type of physical movement required. *Comments:*	☐	☐	☐	
3. Identify the potential need for assistive equipment. *Comments:*	☐	☐	☐	
4. Identify any unusual risks to safe lifting. *Comments:*	☐	☐	☐	
5. Explain the steps required to achieve the goal of safe lifting with the client. *Comments:*	☐	☐	☐	
Planning/Expected Outcomes				
1. Clients will be safely lifted by staff. *Comments:*	☐	☐	☐	
2. Accidents during lifting of clients will be avoided. *Comments:*	☐	☐	☐	
3. Heavy lifting will be facilitated by mechanical devices and a team effort. *Comments:*	☐	☐	☐	
4. Clients and families will be taught safe lifting techniques. *Comments:*	☐	☐	☐	

                    continued on the following page

continued from the previous page

Procedure 38-1	Able to Perform	Able to Perform with Assistance	Unable to Perform	Initials and Date
5. The nurse will practice safe lifting and proper body mechanics. *Comments:*	☐	☐	☐	
Implementation				
1. Wash hands. *Comments:*	☐	☐	☐	
2. Assess the area for obstacles. Reduce or remove safety hazards prior to lifting the client or object. *Comments:*	☐	☐	☐	
3. Assess the area for slippery surfaces. Resolve the slippery surface prior to lifting the client or object. *Comments:*	☐	☐	☐	
4. Assess the area for hidden risks. *Comments:*	☐	☐	☐	
5. Maintain a low center of gravity by bending at the hips and knees, not at the waist. Squat down rather than bend over to lift and lower. *Comments:*	☐	☐	☐	
6. Establish a wide support base with feet spread apart. *Comments:*	☐	☐	☐	
7. Use feet to move, not a twisting or bending motion from the waist. *Comments:*	☐	☐	☐	
8. When pushing or pulling, stand near the object and stagger one foot partially ahead of the other. *Comments:*	☐	☐	☐	
9. When pushing an object, lean into it and apply continuous light pressure. When pulling an object, lean away and grasp with light pressure. Never jerk or twist your body to force a weight to move. *Comments:*	☐	☐	☐	

Procedure 38-1	Able to Perform	Able to Perform with Assistance	Unable to Perform	Initials and Date
10. When stooping to move an object, maintain a wide base of support with feet, flex knees to lower, and maintain straight upper body. *Comments:*	☐	☐	☐	
11. When lifting an object, squat down in front of the object, take a firm hold, and assume a standing position by using the leg muscles, keeping the back straight. *Comments:*	☐	☐	☐	
12. When raising up from a squatting position, arch your back slightly. Keep the buttocks and abdomen tucked in and raise up with your head first. *Comments:*	☐	☐	☐	
13. When lifting or carrying heavy objects, keep the weight as close to your center of gravity as possible. *Comments:*	☐	☐	☐	
14. When reaching for an object, keep the back straight. *Comments:*	☐	☐	☐	
15. Use safety aids and equipment. *Comments:*	☐	☐	☐	

_____   _____

Faculty Signature   Date

Checklist for Procedure 38-2   Turning and Positioning a Client

Name _____ Date _____

School _____

Instructor _____

Course _____

Procedure 38-2 Turning and Positioning a Client	Able to Perform	Able to Perform with Assistance	Unable to Perform	Initials and Date
Assessment				
1. Assess the client's ability to move independently. *Comments:*	☐	☐	☐	
2. Assess the client's flexibility. *Comments:*	☐	☐	☐	
3. Assess the client's overall condition. *Comments:*	☐	☐	☐	
4. Assess the orders for restrictions regarding client positioning. *Comments:*	☐	☐	☐	
Planning/Expected Outcomes				
1. The client will maintain skin integrity. *Comments:*	☐	☐	☐	
2. The client will be comfortable. *Comments:*	☐	☐	☐	
Implementation				
1. Wash hands. *Comments:*	☐	☐	☐	
2. Explain procedure to client. *Comments:*	☐	☐	☐	
3. Gather all necessary equipment. *Comments:*	☐	☐	☐	

     continued on the following page

212 • Checklist – Turning and Positioning a Client

continued from the previous page

Procedure 38-2	Able to Perform	Able to Perform with Assistance	Unable to Perform	Initials and Date
4. Secure adequate assistance to safely complete task. *Comments:*	☐	☐	☐	
5. Adjust bed to comfortable working height. Lower side rail. *Comments:*	☐	☐	☐	
6. Follow proper body mechanics guidelines. *Comments:*	☐	☐	☐	
7. Position drains, tubes, and IVs to accommodate new client position. *Comments:*	☐	☐	☐	
8. Place or assist client into appropriate starting position. *Comments:*	☐	☐	☐	
Moving from Supine to Side-Lying Position 9. Move the client to one side of the bed by lifting the client's body toward you. Roll the client to side-lying position. *Comments:*	☐	☐	☐	
Maintaining Side-Lying Position 10. Follow steps 1 through 8. *Comments:*	☐	☐	☐	
11. Pillows may be placed to support the client. *Comments:*	☐	☐	☐	
Moving from Side-Lying to Prone Position 12. Repeat steps 1 through 8. *Comments:*	☐	☐	☐	
13. Remove positioning support devices. Move the client's inside arm next to the body. Roll the client onto the stomach. Place pillows as needed. *Comments:*	☐	☐	☐	
Maintaining Prone Position 14. Pillows or a folded towel may be used to support the client. *Comments:*	☐	☐	☐	

Procedure 38-2	Able to Perform	Able to Perform with Assistance	Unable to Perform	Initials and Date
Moving from Prone to Supine Position 15. Repeat steps 1 through 8. *Comments:*	☐	☐	☐	
16. Remove supporting devices. Move the client to one side of the bed. Log roll the client toward you. *Comments:*	☐	☐	☐	
Maintaining the Supine Position 17. Pillows, a footboard, heel protectors, or a trochanter roll may be used to support the client. *Comments:*	☐	☐	☐	
18. Replace side rails to upright position and lower the bed. *Comments:*	☐	☐	☐	
19. Place call light within reach of the client. *Comments:*	☐	☐	☐	
20. Place items of frequent use within reach of the client. *Comments:*	☐	☐	☐	
21. Wash hands. *Comments:*	☐	☐	☐	

_____   _____

Faculty Signature　　　　　　　　　　　　　　　　　　　　　　Date

Checklist for Procedure 38-3   Administering Passive Range of Motion (ROM) Exercises

Name _____ Date _____

School _____

Instructor _____

Course _____

Procedure 38-3 Administering Passive Range of Motion (ROM) Exercises	Able to Perform	Able to Perform with Assistance	Unable to Perform	Initials and Date
Assessment				
1. Be aware of the client's medical diagnosis. Comments:	☐	☐	☐	
2. Familiarize yourself with the client's current range of motion. Comments:	☐	☐	☐	
3. Assess client consciousness and cognitive function. Comments:	☐	☐	☐	
Planning/Expected Outcomes				
1. Client will maintain or improve current functional joint mobility. Comments:	☐	☐	☐	
2. Client will regain or improve strength and movement in involved area(s). Comments:	☐	☐	☐	
3. Client will avoid complications of immobility. Comments:	☐	☐	☐	
Implementation				
1. Wash hands and wear gloves. Comments:	☐	☐	☐	
2. Explain procedure to client. Comments:	☐	☐	☐	
3. Provide for privacy, exposing only the extremity to be exercised. Comments:	☐	☐	☐	

     continued on the following page

continued from the previous page

Procedure 38-3	Able to Perform	Able to Perform with Assistance	Unable to Perform	Initials and Date
4. Adjust bed to comfortable height for performing ROM. *Comments:*	☐	☐	☐	
5. Lower bed rail only on the side you are working. *Comments:*	☐	☐	☐	
6. Describe the passive ROM exercises you are performing. *Comments:*	☐	☐	☐	
7. Start at the client's head and perform ROM exercises down each side of the body. *Comments:*	☐	☐	☐	
8. Repeat each ROM exercise as the client tolerates to a maximum of five times. *Comments:*	☐	☐	☐	
9. Head With the client in a sitting position, if possible. • Rotation: Turn the head from side to side. • Flexion and extension: Tilt the head toward the chest and then slightly upward. • Lateral flexion: Tilt the head on each side so as to almost touch the ear to the shoulder. *Comments:*	☐	☐	☐	
10. Neck With the client in a sitting position, if possible. • Rotation: Rotate the neck in a semicircle while supporting the head. *Comments:*	☐	☐	☐	
11. Trunk With the client in a sitting position, if possible. • Flexion and extension: Bend the trunk forward, straighten, and then extend slightly backward. • Rotation: Turn the shoulders forward and return to normal position. • Lateral flexion: Tip trunk to the left side, straighten, tip to the right side. *Comments:*	☐	☐	☐	

Procedure 38-3	Able to Perform	Able to Perform with Assistance	Unable to Perform	Initials and Date

12. Arm
  • Flexion and extension: Extend a straight arm upward toward the head, then downward along the side.
  • Adduction and abduction: Extend a straight arm toward the midline and away from the midline.
  Comments:
	☐	☐	☐	

13. Shoulder
  • Internal and external rotation: Bend the elbow at a 90° angle with upper arm parallel to the shoulder. Move the lower arm upward and downward.
  Comments:
	☐	☐	☐	

14. Elbow
  • Flexion and extension: Supporting the arm, flex and extend the elbow.
  • Pronation and supination: Flex elbow, move the hand in a palm-up and palm-down position.
  Comments:
	☐	☐	☐	

15. Wrist
  • Flexion and extension: Supporting the wrist, flex and extend the wrist.
  • Adduction and abduction: Supporting the lower arm, turn wrist right to left, left to right, then rotate the wrist in a circular motion.
  Comments:
	☐	☐	☐	

16. Hand
  • Flexion and extension: Support the wrist, flex and extend the fingers.
  • Adduction and abduction: Support the wrist, spread fingers apart and then bring them close together.
  • Opposition: Supporting the wrist, touch each finger with the tip of the thumb.
  • Thumb rotation: Support the wrist, rotate the thumb in a circular manner.
  Comments:
	☐	☐	☐	

17. Hip and leg
  With the client in a supine position, if possible.
  • Flexion and extension: Support the lower leg, flex the leg toward the chest and then extend the leg.
  • Internal and external rotation: Support the lower leg, angle the foot inward and outward.
  • Adduction and abduction: Slide the leg away from the client's midline and then back to the midline.
  Comments:
	☐	☐	☐	

     continued on the following page

continued from the previous page

Procedure 38-3	Able to Perform	Able to Perform with Assistance	Unable to Perform	Initials and Date
18. Knee • Flexion and extension: Support the lower leg, flex and extend the knee. *Comments:*	☐	☐	☐	
19. Ankle • Flexion and extension: Support the lower leg, flex and extend the ankle. *Comments:*	☐	☐	☐	
20. Foot • Adduction and abduction: Support the ankle, spread the toes apart and then bring them close together. • Flexion and extension: Support the ankle, extend the toes upward and then flex the toes downward. *Comments:*	☐	☐	☐	
21. Observe client for signs of exertion, pain, or fatigue. *Comments:*	☐	☐	☐	
22. Replace covers and position client in proper body alignment. *Comments:*	☐	☐	☐	
23. Place side rails in original position. *Comments:*	☐	☐	☐	
24. Place call light within reach. *Comments:*	☐	☐	☐	
25. Wash hands. *Comments:*	☐	☐	☐	

_____   _____
Faculty Signature   Date

Checklist for Procedure 38-4   Moving a Client in Bed

Name _____ Date _____

School _____

Instructor _____

Course _____

Procedure 38-4 Moving a Client in Bed	Able to Perform	Able to Perform with Assistance	Unable to Perform	Initials and Date
Assessment				
1. Assess the client's ability to assist with repositioning. *Comments:*	☐	☐	☐	
2. Assess the client's ability to understand and follow directions. *Comments:*	☐	☐	☐	
3. Assess the client's environment. *Comments:*	☐	☐	☐	
Planning/Expected Outcomes				
1. The client will be moved in bed without injury. *Comments:*	☐	☐	☐	
2. The client will be moved in bed without injury to the staff. *Comments:*	☐	☐	☐	
3. The client will report an increase in comfort. *Comments:*	☐	☐	☐	
4. All tubes, lines, and drains will remain patent and intact. *Comments:*	☐	☐	☐	
Implementation				
Moving a Client Up in Bed with One Nurse 1. Wash hands. *Comments:*	☐	☐	☐	
2. Inform client of reason for the move. *Comments:*	☐	☐	☐	

                    continued on the following page

continued from the previous page

Procedure 38-4	Able to Perform	Able to Perform with Assistance	Unable to Perform	Initials and Date
3. Elevate bed. Lower head of bed. Lower side rails. *Comments:*	☐	☐	☐	
4. Place pillow against the headboard. *Comments:*	☐	☐	☐	
5. Have the client fold arms across the chest, if no overhead trapeze is present. *Comments:*	☐	☐	☐	
6. Have client hold on to the overhead trapeze. *Comments:*	☐	☐	☐	
7. Have the client bend knees and place feet flat on the bed. *Comments:*	☐	☐	☐	
8. Stand at head of the bed, feet apart, knees bent. *Comments:*	☐	☐	☐	
9. Slide one hand and arm under the client's shoulder, the other under the client's thigh. *Comments:*	☐	☐	☐	
10. Lift the client while client pushes with the legs. *Comments:*	☐	☐	☐	
11. If available, have the client pull up using the trapeze as you move the client. *Comments:*	☐	☐	☐	
12. Repeat these steps until the client is high enough in bed. *Comments:*	☐	☐	☐	
13. Return the client's pillow under the head. *Comments:*	☐	☐	☐	
14. Elevate head of bed, if tolerated by client. *Comments:*	☐	☐	☐	

Procedure 38-4	Able to Perform	Able to Perform with Assistance	Unable to Perform	Initials and Date
15. Assess client for comfort. *Comments:*	☐	☐	☐	
16. Adjust the client's bedclothes as needed for comfort. *Comments:*	☐	☐	☐	
17. Lower bed and elevate side rails. *Comments:*	☐	☐	☐	
18. Wash hands. *Comments:*	☐	☐	☐	
Moving a Client Up in Bed with Two or More Nurses 19. Wash hands and apply gloves if needed. *Comments:*	☐	☐	☐	
20. Inform client of reason for the move. *Comments:*	☐	☐	☐	
21. Elevate bed. Lower head of bed. Lower side rails. *Comments:*	☐	☐	☐	
22. Place turn/draw sheet under client's back and head. *Comments:*	☐	☐	☐	
23. Roll up the draw sheet on each side until it is next to the client. *Comments:*	☐	☐	☐	
24. Follow steps 4 through 7. *Comments:*	☐	☐	☐	
25. The nurses stand on either side of the bed, with knees flexed, feet apart in a wide stance. *Comments:*	☐	☐	☐	
26. The nurses hold their elbows close to their bodies. *Comments:*	☐	☐	☐	

continued on the following page

continued from the previous page

Procedure 38-4	Able to Perform	Able to Perform with Assistance	Unable to Perform	Initials and Date
27. At the signal to move, lift up and forward in one smooth motion. *Comments:*	☐	☐	☐	
28. Repeat until the client is high enough in bed. *Comments:*	☐	☐	☐	
29. Return the client's pillow under his head. *Comments:*	☐	☐	☐	
30. Elevate head of bed, if tolerated by client. *Comments:*	☐	☐	☐	
31. Assess client for comfort. *Comments:*	☐	☐	☐	
32. Adjust the client's bedclothes for comfort. *Comments:*	☐	☐	☐	
33. Lower bed and elevate side rails. *Comments:*	☐	☐	☐	
34. Wash hands. *Comments:*	☐	☐	☐	

_____   _____

Faculty Signature   Date

Checklist for Procedure 38-5 Log Rolling a Client

Name _____ Date _____

School _____

Instructor _____

Course _____

Procedure 38-5 Log Rolling a Client	Able to Perform	Able to Perform with Assistance	Unable to Perform	Initials and Date
Assessment				
1. Assess the client's ability to assist in log rolling. *Comments:*	☐	☐	☐	
2. Assess the client's flexibility. *Comments:*	☐	☐	☐	
3. Assess the client's overall condition. *Comments:*	☐	☐	☐	
4. Assess orders that restrict client positioning or movement. *Comments:*	☐	☐	☐	
Planning/Expected Outcomes				
1. The client will maintain proper body alignment. *Comments:*	☐	☐	☐	
2. The client will be comfortable. *Comments:*	☐	☐	☐	
3. The client will be turned as a unit without sustaining injury. *Comments:*	☐	☐	☐	
Implementation				
1. Wash hands and apply gloves. *Comments:*	☐	☐	☐	
2. Inform the client of the reason and need for turning. *Comments:*	☐	☐	☐	

                    continued on the following page

continued from the previous page

Procedure 38-5	Able to Perform	Able to Perform with Assistance	Unable to Perform	Initials and Date
3. Elevate the bed to a working height. *Comments:*	☐	☐	☐	
4. Using one or more assistants, place a turn sheet under the client. *Comments:*	☐	☐	☐	
5. The lead nurse provides directions for the client and the other nurses. *Comments:*	☐	☐	☐	
6. With one staff member on each side of the bed: • The lead nurse gives the signal for the move. • The staff member on the side of the bed holds the turn/draw sheet to guide the direction of the move. • The second staff member applies gentle pressure at the client's back in the direction of the move, using the draw sheet. • The client assists with the turning as much as possible. *Comments:*	☐	☐	☐	
7. Position pillows at the client's back and abdomen. *Comments:*	☐	☐	☐	
8. Assess for client's comfort and proper body alignment. *Comments:*	☐	☐	☐	
9. Elevate side rails and lower the bed height. *Comments:*	☐	☐	☐	
10. This procedure can be repeated for turning the client to the supine position. *Comments:*	☐	☐	☐	

Faculty Signature   Date

Checklist for Procedure 38-6　Assisting from Bed to Wheelchair, Commode, or Chair

Name _____ Date _____

School _____

Instructor _____

Course _____

Procedure 38-6 **Assisting from Bed to Wheelchair, Commode, or Chair**	Able to Perform	Able to Perform with Assistance	Unable to Perform	Initials and Date
Assessment				
1. Assess the client's current level of mobility. *Comments:*	☐	☐	☐	
2. Assess for any impediments to mobility. *Comments:*	☐	☐	☐	
3. Assess the client's level of understanding and anxiety regarding the procedure. *Comments:*	☐	☐	☐	
4. Assess the client's environment. *Comments:*	☐	☐	☐	
5. Assess the equipment. *Comments:*	☐	☐	☐	
Planning/Expected Outcomes				
1. The client will be transferred without pain or injury. *Comments:*	☐	☐	☐	
2. Drainage tubes, IVs, or other devices will be intact. *Comments:*	☐	☐	☐	
3. The client's skin will be intact and undamaged. *Comments:*	☐	☐	☐	
Implementation				
1. Inform client about desired purpose and destination. *Comments:*	☐	☐	☐	

　　　　continued on the following page

continued from the previous page

Procedure 38-6	Able to Perform	Able to Perform with Assistance	Unable to Perform	Initials and Date
2. Assess client for ability to assist with and understand the transfer. *Comments:*	☐	☐	☐	
3. Lock the bed in position. *Comments:*	☐	☐	☐	
4. Place any splints, braces, or other devices on the client. *Comments:*	☐	☐	☐	
5. Place shoes or slippers on the client's feet. *Comments:*	☐	☐	☐	
6. Lower the height of the bed to lowest possible position. *Comments:*	☐	☐	☐	
7. Slowly raise the head of the bed if this is not contraindicated. *Comments:*	☐	☐	☐	
8. Place an arm under the client's legs and behind the client's back. Pivot the client so he is sitting on the edge of the bed. *Comments:*	☐	☐	☐	
9. Allow client to dangle for 2 to 5 minutes. *Comments:*	☐	☐	☐	
10. Place the chair or wheelchair at a 45° angle close to the bed. *Comments:*	☐	☐	☐	
11. Lock wheelchair brakes and elevate the foot pedals. *Comments:*	☐	☐	☐	
12. Place gait belt around the client's waist, if needed. *Comments:*	☐	☐	☐	

Procedure 38-6	Able to Perform	Able to Perform with Assistance	Unable to Perform	Initials and Date
13. Assist client to side of bed until feet are firmly on the floor and slightly apart. *Comments:*	☐	☐	☐	
14. Grasp the sides of the gait belt or place your hands just below the client's axilla. Bend your knees and assist the client to a standing position. *Comments:*	☐	☐	☐	
15. Standing close to the client, pivot until the client's back is toward the chair. *Comments:*	☐	☐	☐	
16. Have client place hands on the arm supports. *Comments:*	☐	☐	☐	
17. Bend at the knees, easing the client into a sitting position. *Comments:*	☐	☐	☐	
18. Assist client to maintain proper posture. *Comments:*	☐	☐	☐	
19. Secure the safety belt, place client's feet on foot pedals, and release brakes to move client. If the client is sitting in a chair, offer a footstool. *Comments:*	☐	☐	☐	
20. Wash hands. *Comments:*	☐	☐	☐	

_____   _____

Faculty Signature   Date

Checklist for Procedure 38-7　Assisting from Bed to Stretcher

Name _____　Date _____

School _____

Instructor _____

Course _____

Procedure 38-7 Assisting from Bed to Stretcher	Able to Perform	Able to Perform with Assistance	Unable to Perform	Initials and Date
Assessment				
1. Assess the client's current level of mobility. *Comments:*	☐	☐	☐	
2. Assess for injury. *Comments:*	☐	☐	☐	
3. Assess for any impediments to mobility. *Comments:*	☐	☐	☐	
4. Assess the client's level of understanding. *Comments:*	☐	☐	☐	
5. Assess the client's environment. *Comments:*	☐	☐	☐	
6. Make sure the stretcher is safe to use. *Comments:*	☐	☐	☐	
Planning/Expected Outcomes				
1. The client will be transferred without pain or injury. *Comments:*	☐	☐	☐	
2. Drainage tubes, IVs, or other devices will remain intact. *Comments:*	☐	☐	☐	
3. The client's skin will be intact and undamaged. *Comments:*	☐	☐	☐	
Implementation				
Transferring a Client with Minimum Assistance 1. Inform client about desired purpose and destination. *Comments:*	☐	☐	☐	

　　　continued on the following page

continued from the previous page

Procedure 38-7	Able to Perform	Able to Perform with Assistance	Unable to Perform	Initials and Date
2. Raise the bed 1 inch higher than the stretcher, and lock brakes of bed and stretcher. *Comments:*	☐	☐	☐	
3. Instruct client to move close to stretcher. Lower side rails of bed and stretcher. *Comments:*	☐	☐	☐	
4. Stand at outer side of stretcher and push it toward bed. *Comments:*	☐	☐	☐	
5. Instruct client to move onto stretcher. Assist as needed. *Comments:*	☐	☐	☐	
6. Cover client with sheet or bath blanket. *Comments:*	☐	☐	☐	
7. Elevate side rails on stretcher and secure safety belts. Release brakes of stretcher. *Comments:*	☐	☐	☐	
8. Stand at head of stretcher to guide it when pushing. *Comments:*	☐	☐	☐	
9. Wash hands. *Comments:*	☐	☐	☐	
Transferring a Client with Maximum Assistance 10. Repeat steps 1 and 2. *Comments:*	☐	☐	☐	
11. Assess amount of assistance required for transfer. *Comments:*	☐	☐	☐	
12. Lock wheels of bed and stretcher. *Comments:*	☐	☐	☐	
13. Have one nurse stand close to client's head. *Comments:*	☐	☐	☐	

Procedure 38-7	Able to Perform	Able to Perform with Assistance	Unable to Perform	Initials and Date
14. Log roll the client and place a lift sheet under the client. *Comments:*	☐	☐	☐	
15. Empty all drainage bags. Record amounts. Secure drainage system to client's gown. *Comments:*	☐	☐	☐	
16. Move client to edge of bed near stretcher. *Comments:*	☐	☐	☐	
17. Have the nurse on the nonstretcher side of bed hold the stretcher side of the lift sheet up to prevent the client from falling. *Comments:*	☐	☐	☐	
18. Place pillow or slider board overlapping the bed and stretcher. *Comments:*	☐	☐	☐	
19. Have staff members grasp edges of lift sheet. *Comments:*	☐	☐	☐	
20. On the count of three, staff members pull lift sheet and the client onto the stretcher. *Comments:*	☐	☐	☐	
21. Position client on stretcher. Cover with a sheet or bath blanket. *Comments:*	☐	☐	☐	
22. Secure safety belts and elevate side rails of stretcher. *Comments:*	☐	☐	☐	
23. Move IV from bed pole to stretcher IV pole after client transfer, if indicated. *Comments:*	☐	☐	☐	
24. Wash hands. *Comments:*	☐	☐	☐	

_____   _____

Faculty Signature   Date

Checklist for Procedure 38-8   Using a Hydraulic Lift

Name _____ Date _____

School _____

Instructor _____

Course _____

Procedure 38-8 Using a Hydraulic Lift	Able to Perform	Able to Perform with Assistance	Unable to Perform	Initials and Date
Assessment				
1. Identify clients with any injuries of the vertebrae. *Comments:*	☐	☐	☐	
2. Identify any equipment that is connected to the client. *Comments:*	☐	☐	☐	
3. Assess client's need for transfer, and physical and mental condition. *Comments:*	☐	☐	☐	
4. Assess client's ability to assist and understand transfer. *Comments:*	☐	☐	☐	
5. Assess number of staff needed for transfer. *Comments:*	☐	☐	☐	
6. Determine whether client is in appropriate clothes and ready for transfer. *Comments:*	☐	☐	☐	
Planning/Expected Outcomes				
1. Client will be transferred safely. *Comments:*	☐	☐	☐	
2. Client will not experience anxiety during the transfer. *Comments:*	☐	☐	☐	
3. Client will incur no injuries. *Comments:*	☐	☐	☐	
4. Privacy will be maintained. *Comments:*	☐	☐	☐	

                    continued on the following page

continued from the previous page

Procedure 38-8	Able to Perform	Able to Perform with Assistance	Unable to Perform	Initials and Date
Implementation				
1. Wash hands. *Comments:*	☐	☐	☐	
2. Check the orders to determine the length of time the client may sit. *Comments:*	☐	☐	☐	
3. Determine the client's medical diagnosis and any other problems. *Comments:*	☐	☐	☐	
4. Ask the client how long ago he or she last sat. *Comments:*	☐	☐	☐	
5. Lock the wheels of the bed. *Comments:*	☐	☐	☐	
6. Position the chair close to the bed. *Comments:*	☐	☐	☐	
7. Position drainage bags and tubing on the chair side of the bed. *Comments:*	☐	☐	☐	
8. Clamp and disconnect any tubing if permitted. *Comments:*	☐	☐	☐	
9. Roll the client on her side and position the sling beside the client. *Comments:*	☐	☐	☐	
10. Roll the client on the other side, pull the sling through, and position the sling on the bed. *Comments:*	☐	☐	☐	
11. Roll the client back onto the sling and fold arms over the chest. *Comments:*	☐	☐	☐	
12. Make sure the sling is centered. *Comments:*	☐	☐	☐	

Procedure 38-8	Able to Perform	Able to Perform with Assistance	Unable to Perform	Initials and Date
13. Lower the side rail. Position the lift on the chair side of the bed. Spread the base of the hydraulic lift. *Comments:*	☐	☐	☐	
14. Lift the frame and pass it over the client. Lower the frame and attach the hooks to the sling. *Comments:*	☐	☐	☐	
15. Raise the client from the bed by pumping the handle. *Comments:*	☐	☐	☐	
16. Secure the client with a safety belt and cover with a blanket. *Comments:*	☐	☐	☐	
17. Steer the client away from the bed and slide a chair through the base of the lift. *Comments:*	☐	☐	☐	
18. Lower the client into the chair and disconnect the sling from the lift. *Comments:*	☐	☐	☐	
19. Reposition and reconnect tubing as necessary. *Comments:*	☐	☐	☐	
20. Assess how well the client tolerated the move. *Comments:*	☐	☐	☐	
21. Place call button within reach, see to client's comfort, and apply restraints if needed. *Comments:*	☐	☐	☐	
22. Reverse the procedure to return the client to the bed. *Comments:*	☐	☐	☐	
23. Wash hands. *Comments:*	☐	☐	☐	

_____　　　_____

Faculty Signature　　　　　　　　　　　　　　　　　　Date

Checklist for Procedure 38-9 Assisting with Ambulation and Safe Falling

Name _____ Date _____

School _____

Instructor _____

Course _____

Procedure 38-9 Assisting with Ambulation and Safe Falling	Able to Perform	Able to Perform with Assistance	Unable to Perform	Initials and Date
Assessment				
1. Determine the client's most recent activity level and tolerance. *Comments:*	☐	☐	☐	
2. Assess the client's condition. *Comments:*	☐	☐	☐	
3. Check for handrails, a clean and level floor, and adequate lighting. *Comments:*	☐	☐	☐	
4. Assess the client's ambulation equipment. *Comments:*	☐	☐	☐	
5. Check the client's clothing. *Comments:*	☐	☐	☐	
6. While the client is ambulating, assess client's gait and bearing. *Comments:*	☐	☐	☐	
7. After ambulation, assess the client's ability to recover from the activity. *Comments:*	☐	☐	☐	
Planning/Expected Outcomes				
1. The client will be able to walk a predetermined distance, with assistance as needed, and return to the starting point. *Comments:*	☐	☐	☐	
2. While walking, the client will not suffer any injury. *Comments:*	☐	☐	☐	

continued on the following page

continued from the previous page

Procedure 38-9	Able to Perform	Able to Perform with Assistance	Unable to Perform	Initials and Date
3. The client will be able to increase the distance he can walk and/or will require less assistance to accomplish the distance. *Comments:*	☐	☐	☐	

Implementation

1. Move IV infusions from the existing location to a position closer to the client. If IV infusion pole is portable, place the pole near the client on the same side of the bed or chair. If infusion pump is not portable or the client does not have a rolling IV pole, secure an IV pole. Remove IV fluids that are infusing via infusion pump only if medical condition or fluids are compatible with gravity flow. Regulate any IV fluids via gravity flow immediately. *Comments:*	☐	☐	☐	
2. Transfer the IV infusion from the bed IV pole to the portable IV pole. *Comments:*	☐	☐	☐	
3. Empty the drainage bag, if present, prior to ambulation. Remove the urinary drainage bag from the bed. *Comments:*	☐	☐	☐	
4. When the client has a drainage tube, be sure to secure the drainage tube and bag prior to ambulation. *Comments:*	☐	☐	☐	
5. Ambulating the client with a closed chest tube drainage system often requires two nurses. Remove the drainage system from the bed. Hold the closed chest tube drainage system upright at all times to maintain the water seal. *Comments:*	☐	☐	☐	
6. Use a transfer belt or gait belt when ambulating a client who is weak. *Comments:*	☐	☐	☐	
7. If a client feels faint or dizzy during dangling, return the client to a supine position in bed and lower the head of the bed. Assess the client's blood pressure and pulse. *Comments:*	☐	☐	☐	

Procedure 38-9	Able to Perform	Able to Perform with Assistance	Unable to Perform	Initials and Date
8. If the client feels faint or dizzy during ambulation, allow the client to sit in a chair. Stay with the client for safety. Request another nurse to secure a wheelchair to return the client to bed. *Comments:*	☐	☐	☐	
9. If the client feels faint or dizzy during the ambulation and starts to fall, ease the client to the floor while supporting and protecting the client's head. Ask other personnel to assist you in returning the client to bed. Assess orthostatic blood pressures. *Comments:*	☐	☐	☐	
Safe Walking 1. Inform client of the purposes and distance of the walking exercise. *Comments:*	☐	☐	☐	
2. Elevate the head of the bed and wait several minutes. *Comments:*	☐	☐	☐	
3. Lower the bed height. *Comments:*	☐	☐	☐	
4. With one arm on the client's back and one arm under the client's upper legs, move the client into the dangling position. *Comments:*	☐	☐	☐	
5. Have the client dangle for several minutes. *Comments:*	☐	☐	☐	
6. Assist client in putting on slippers or other nonskid or nonslip shoes. *Comments:*	☐	☐	☐	
7. Place gait belt around client's waist; secure the buckle in front. *Comments:*	☐	☐	☐	

  continued on the following page

continued from the previous page

Procedure 38-9	Able to Perform	Able to Perform with Assistance	Unable to Perform	Initials and Date
8. Stand in front of client with your knees touching client's knees. *Comments:*	☐	☐	☐	
9. Place arms under client's axilla. *Comments:*	☐	☐	☐	
10. Assist client to a standing position, allowing client time to balance. *Comments:*	☐	☐	☐	
11. Help the client ambulate. *Comments:*	☐	☐	☐	
12. Assist the client back to the bed or chair. Make the client comfortable, and make sure all lines and tubes are secure. *Comments:*	☐	☐	☐	
13. Secure bed in lowest position, elevate side rails, and place all client's personal items within easy reach. *Comments:*	☐	☐	☐	
14. Document the activity. *Comments:*	☐	☐	☐	
15. Wash hands. *Comments:*	☐	☐	☐	

Faculty Signature _____   Date _____

Checklist for Procedure 38-10   Assisting with Crutches, Cane, or Walker

Name _____ Date _____

School _____

Instructor _____

Course _____

Procedure 38-10 **Assisting with Crutches, Cane, or Walker**	Able to Perform	Able to Perform with Assistance	Unable to Perform	Initials and Date
Assessment				
1. Assess the reason the client requires an assistive device. *Comments:*	☐	☐	☐	
2. Assess the client's physical limitations. *Comments:*	☐	☐	☐	
3. Assess the client's physical environment. *Comments:*	☐	☐	☐	
4. Assess the client's ability to understand and follow directions. *Comments:*	☐	☐	☐	
Planning/Expected Outcomes				
1. The client will ambulate safely with an assistive device. *Comments:*	☐	☐	☐	
2. The client will feel confident while using the assistive device. *Comments:*	☐	☐	☐	
Implementation				
Crutch Walking				
1. Inform client you will be teaching crutch ambulation. *Comments:*	☐	☐	☐	
2. Assess client for strength, mobility, range of motion, visual acuity, perceptual difficulties, and balance. *Comments:*	☐	☐	☐	

          continued on the following page

continued from the previous page

Procedure 38-10	Able to Perform	Able to Perform with Assistance	Unable to Perform	Initials and Date
3. Adjust crutches to fit the client. • The crutch pad should fit 1.5 to 2 inches below the axilla. • The hand grip should keep the elbows bent at 30° flexion. *Comments:*	☐	☐	☐	
4. Lower the height of the bed. *Comments:*	☐	☐	☐	
5. Dangle the client. Assess for vertigo. *Comments:*	☐	☐	☐	
6. Instruct client to position crutches lateral to and forward of feet. Demonstrate correct positioning. *Comments:*	☐	☐	☐	
7. Apply the gait belt around the client's waist if needed. *Comments:*	☐	☐	☐	
8. Assist the client to a standing position with crutches. *Comments:*	☐	☐	☐	
Four-Point Gait 9. • Position crutches to the side and in front of each foot. • Move the right crutch forward 4 to 6 inches. • Move the left foot forward, even with the left crutch. • Move the left crutch forward 4 to 6 inches. • Move the right foot forward, even with the right crutch. • Repeat the four-point gait. *Comments:*	☐	☐	☐	
Three-Point Gait 10. • Advance both crutches and the weaker leg forward together. • Move the stronger leg forward, even with the crutches. • Repeat the three-point gait. *Comments:*	☐	☐	☐	

Procedure 38-10	Able to Perform	Able to Perform with Assistance	Unable to Perform	Initials and Date

Two-Point Gait
11. • Move the left crutch and right leg forward 4 to 6 inches.
   • Move the right crutch and left leg forward 4 to 6 inches.
   • Repeat the two-point gait.
Comments:
	☐	☐	☐	

Swing-Through Gait
12. • Move both crutches forward together 4 to 6 inches.
   • Move both legs forward, even with the crutches.
   • Repeat the swing-through gait.
Comments:
	☐	☐	☐	

Walking Up Stairs
13. • Instruct client to position the crutches as if walking.
   • Place the strong leg on the first step.
   • Pull the weak leg up and move the crutches up to the first step.
   • Repeat for all steps.
Comments:
	☐	☐	☐	

Walking Down Stairs
14. • Position the crutches as if walking.
   • Place weight on the strong leg.
   • Move the crutches down to the next lower step.
   • Place partial weight on hands and crutches.
   • Move the weak leg down to the step with the crutches.
   • Put total weight on arms and crutches.
   • Move strong leg to same step as weak leg and crutches.
   • Repeat for all steps.
Comments:
	☐	☐	☐	

15. Set realistic goals. *Comments:*	☐	☐	☐	
16. Consult with a physical therapist. *Comments:*	☐	☐	☐	
17. Wash hands. *Comments:*	☐	☐	☐	
Walking with a Cane 18. Inform client you will be teaching cane ambulation. *Comments:*	☐	☐	☐	

continued on the following page

continued from the previous page

Procedure 38-10	Able to Perform	Able to Perform with Assistance	Unable to Perform	Initials and Date
19. Lower the height of the bed. *Comments:*	☐	☐	☐	
20. Dangle the client. Assess for vertigo. *Comments:*	☐	☐	☐	
21. Assess client for strength, mobility, range of motion, visual acuity, perceptual difficulties, and balance. *Comments:*	☐	☐	☐	
22. Apply the gait belt around the client's waist, if needed. *Comments:*	☐	☐	☐	
23. Have the client hold the cane in the hand opposite the affected leg. *Comments:*	☐	☐	☐	
24. Have the client push up from sitting while pushing down on the bed with the arms. *Comments:*	☐	☐	☐	
25. Have the client stand at the bedside for a few moments. *Comments:*	☐	☐	☐	
26. Assess the height of the cane. *Comments:*	☐	☐	☐	
27. Walk to the side and slightly behind the client. *Comments:*	☐	☐	☐	
The Cane Gait 28. • Move the cane and the weaker leg forward at the same time for the same distance. • Place weight on the weaker leg and the cane. • Move the strong leg forward. • Place weight on the strong leg. *Comments:*	☐	☐	☐	

Procedure 38-10	Able to Perform	Able to Perform with Assistance	Unable to Perform	Initials and Date
Sitting with a Cane 29. • Have client turn around and back up to the chair. 　• Client grasps the arm of the chair with the free hand and lowers into the chair. 　• Place the cane out of the way but within reach. *Comments:*	☐	☐	☐	
30. Set realistic goals. *Comments:*	☐	☐	☐	
31. Consult with a physical therapist. *Comments:*	☐	☐	☐	
32. Wash hands. *Comments:*	☐	☐	☐	
Walking with a Walker 33. Inform client that you will be teaching walker ambulation. *Comments:*	☐	☐	☐	
34. Lower the height of the bed. *Comments:*	☐	☐	☐	
35. Dangle the client. Assess for vertigo. *Comments:*	☐	☐	☐	
36. Provide a robe and shoes with firm, nonslip soles. *Comments:*	☐	☐	☐	
37. Assess client for strength, mobility, range of motion, visual acuity, perceptual difficulties, and balance. *Comments:*	☐	☐	☐	
38. Apply the gait belt around the client's waist if needed. *Comments:*	☐	☐	☐	
39. Place the walker in front of the client. *Comments:*	☐	☐	☐	
40. Have the client push up from sitting while pushing down on the bed with arms. *Comments:*	☐	☐	☐	

　　　continued on the following page

continued from the previous page

Procedure 38-10	Able to Perform	Able to Perform with Assistance	Unable to Perform	Initials and Date
41. Have the client transfer hands to the walker, one at a time. *Comments:*	☐	☐	☐	
42. The handgrips should be just below waist level. *Comments:*	☐	☐	☐	
43. Walk to the side and slightly behind the client. *Comments:*	☐	☐	☐	
The Walker Gait 44. • Move the walker and weaker leg forward at the same time. • Place as much weight as allowed on the weaker leg. • Move the strong leg forward. • Shift the weight to the strong leg. *Comments:*	☐	☐	☐	
Sitting with a Walker 45. • Have client turn around and back up to the chair. • Have client place hands on the chair armrests, one hand at a time. • Using the armrests for support, client lowers into the chair. *Comments:*	☐	☐	☐	
46. Set realistic goals. *Comments:*	☐	☐	☐	
47. Consult with a physical therapist. *Comments:*	☐	☐	☐	
48. Wash hands. *Comments:*	☐	☐	☐	

Faculty Signature   Date

Checklist for Procedure 39-1   Maintaining and Cleaning the Tracheostomy Tube

Name _____ Date _____

School _____

Instructor _____

Course _____

Procedure 39-1 **Maintaining and Cleaning the Tracheostomy Tube**	Able to Perform	Able to Perform with Assistance	Unable to Perform	Initials and Date
Assessment				
1. Assess respirations for rate, rhythm, and depth. *Comments:*	☐	☐	☐	
2. Auscultate lung fields. *Comments:*	☐	☐	☐	
3. Monitor arterial blood gas and/or pulse oximetry values. *Comments:*	☐	☐	☐	
4. Assess passage of air through tracheostomy tube. *Comments:*	☐	☐	☐	
5. Evaluate amount and color of tracheal secretions. *Comments:*	☐	☐	☐	
6. Assess anxiety, restlessness, and fear. *Comments:*	☐	☐	☐	
7. Assess the client's understanding of the procedure. *Comments:*	☐	☐	☐	
Planning/Expected Outcomes				
1. The tracheostomy site will heal with minimal drainage and erythema. *Comments:*	☐	☐	☐	
2. There will be no evidence of infection. *Comments:*	☐	☐	☐	
3. The client will maintain a patent airway. *Comments:*	☐	☐	☐	

             continued on the following page

continued from the previous page

Procedure 39-1	Able to Perform	Able to Perform with Assistance	Unable to Perform	Initials and Date
4. The inner and outer cannulas will be free of secretions. The ties will be clean and secure. *Comments:*	☐	☐	☐	
Implementation				
Cleaning Trach Tube Site 1. Wash hands and apply gloves. *Comments:*	☐	☐	☐	
2. Remove soiled dressing and discard. *Comments:*	☐	☐	☐	
3. Cleanse neck plate with cotton applicators and hydrogen peroxide. *Comments:*	☐	☐	☐	
4. Rinse neck plate with applicators and sterile water or saline. *Comments:*	☐	☐	☐	
5. Cleanse skin under neck plate with cotton applicators and hydrogen peroxide. *Comments:*	☐	☐	☐	
6. Rinse skin under neck plate with applicators and sterile water or saline. *Comments:*	☐	☐	☐	
7. Dry skin under neck plate with dry cotton applicators. *Comments:*	☐	☐	☐	
One-Person Technique of Changing Tracheostomy Ties 8. Prepare clean tracheostomy ties. • Cut twill tape to fit around the client's neck plus 6 inches. Cut the ends of the tape on the diagonal. • Open Velcro ties on continuous neck band. *Comments:*	☐	☐	☐	
9. Leave the old ties in place. Insert one end of the new tie through the neck plate from back to front. Pull the tie ends even, and bring both ends around the back of the neck to the other side. *Comments:*	☐	☐	☐	

Procedure 39-1	Able to Perform	Able to Perform with Assistance	Unable to Perform	Initials and Date
10. Insert the end of the tape through the second opening of the neck plate from back to front. *Comments:*	☐	☐	☐	
11. Securely tie the two ends of the new tape at side of neck. *Comments:*	☐	☐	☐	
12. Cut and remove old tracheostomy tapes and discard. *Comments:*	☐	☐	☐	
13. Place one finger under tracheostomy ties to test security. *Comments:*	☐	☐	☐	
Two-Person Technique of Changing Tracheostomy Ties 14. Cut two pieces of twill tape about 12 to 14 inches in length. *Comments:*	☐	☐	☐	
15. Fold about 1 inch at the end of twill tape and cut a half-inch slit lengthwise in the center of the fold. Repeat for other tape. *Comments:*	☐	☐	☐	
16. The second person holds the tracheostomy tube in place with fingers on both sides of the neck plate. *Comments:*	☐	☐	☐	
17. Cut old tracheostomy ties and discard. *Comments:*	☐	☐	☐	
18. Insert the split end of the twill tape through the opening on one side of the neck plate. Pull the distal end of the tie through the cut and pull tightly. *Comments:*	☐	☐	☐	
19. Repeat procedure with second piece of twill tape. *Comments:*	☐	☐	☐	
20. Tie tracheostomy tapes securely at the side of the neck. *Comments:*	☐	☐	☐	

                 continued on the following page

continued from the previous page

Procedure 39-1	Able to Perform	Able to Perform with Assistance	Unable to Perform	Initials and Date
21. Insert one finger under tracheostomy tapes. *Comments:*	☐	☐	☐	
22. Insert lint-free tracheostomy gauze under neck plate of tube. *Comments:*	☐	☐	☐	
23. Discard all used materials and wash hands. *Comments:*	☐	☐	☐	

_____

Faculty Signature

_____

Date

Checklist for Procedure 39-2　Suctioning Endotracheal and Tracheal Tubes

Name _____ Date _____

School _____

Instructor _____

Course _____

Procedure 39-2 **Suctioning Endotracheal and Tracheal Tubes**	Able to Perform	Able to Perform with Assistance	Unable to Perform	Initials and Date
Assessment				
1. Assess respirations for rate, rhythm, and depth. *Comments:*	☐	☐	☐	
2. Auscultate lung fields. *Comments:*	☐	☐	☐	
3. Monitor arterial blood gas and/or pulse oximetry values. *Comments:*	☐	☐	☐	
4. Assess passage of air through the endotracheal/tracheal tube. *Comments:*	☐	☐	☐	
5. Monitor secretions for amount, color, consistency, and odor. *Comments:*	☐	☐	☐	
6. Assess for anxiety and restlessness. *Comments:*	☐	☐	☐	
7. Assess the client's understanding of the suctioning procedure. *Comments:*	☐	☐	☐	
Planning/Expected Outcomes				
1. The client will have no crackles or wheezes in large airways and no cyanosis. *Comments:*	☐	☐	☐	
2. The client will appear to breathe comfortably. *Comments:*	☐	☐	☐	
3. The client will have minimal amount of thin secretions. *Comments:*	☐	☐	☐	

　　　　continued on the following page

continued from the previous page

Procedure 39-2	Able to Perform	Able to Perform with Assistance	Unable to Perform	Initials and Date
4. The client will maintain a patent airway. *Comments:*	☐	☐	☐	

Implementation

Suctioning Tracheal Tube

	Able to Perform	Able to Perform with Assistance	Unable to Perform	Initials and Date
1. Assess respirations and breath sounds. *Comments:*	☐	☐	☐	
2. Assemble supplies on bedside table. *Comments:*	☐	☐	☐	
3. Wash hands. *Comments:*	☐	☐	☐	
4. Connect suction tube to source of negative pressure. *Comments:*	☐	☐	☐	
5. Administer oxygen or use Ambu bag. *Comments:*	☐	☐	☐	
6. Remove inner cannula and clean, if reusable, or set aside if disposable. *Comments:*	☐	☐	☐	
7. Apply sterile glove to your dominant hand. *Comments:*	☐	☐	☐	
8. Open sterile suction catheter, remove it from package with your sterile hand, and wrap the catheter around your sterile hand from the tip down to the port end. Or use the reusable closed system catheter. Attach catheter to suction. *Comments:*	☐	☐	☐	
9. Insert the catheter into the trachea without suction. *Comments:*	☐	☐	☐	
10. Apply suction while gently rotating the catheter and removing it. • Disposable catheter: Apply suction by placing your thumb over the open port of the catheter. • Closed system catheter: Apply suction by depressing the white button at the catheter connector. *Comments:*	☐	☐	☐	

Procedure 39-2	Able to Perform	Able to Perform with Assistance	Unable to Perform	Initials and Date
11. Wrap the disposable suction catheter around your sterile hand while withdrawing it from the tube. *Comments:*	☐	☐	☐	
12. Suction for no more than 10 seconds. *Comments:*	☐	☐	☐	
13. Administer oxygen using the ventilator or using an Ambu bag. *Comments:*	☐	☐	☐	
14. Assess airway and repeat suctioning as necessary. *Comments:*	☐	☐	☐	
15. Clean inner cannula or replace disposable inner cannula. *Comments:*	☐	☐	☐	
16. Reinsert inner cannula and lock into place. *Comments:*	☐	☐	☐	
17. Apply humidified oxygen or compressed air. *Comments:*	☐	☐	☐	
18. Remove gloves and discard. *Comments:*	☐	☐	☐	
19. Wash hands. *Comments:*	☐	☐	☐	
20. Record the procedure. *Comments:*	☐	☐	☐	
Suctioning an Endotracheal Tube 21. Repeat steps 1 through 14. *Comments:*	☐	☐	☐	
22. Remove gloves and discard. *Comments:*	☐	☐	☐	

continued on the following page

continued from the previous page

Procedure 39-2	Able to Perform	Able to Perform with Assistance	Unable to Perform	Initials and Date
23. Wash hands. *Comments:*	☐	☐	☐	
24. Record the procedure. *Comments:*	☐	☐	☐	

_____

Faculty Signature

_____

Date

Checklist for Procedure 39-3   Administering Oxygen Therapy

Name _____ Date _____

School _____

Instructor _____

Course _____

Procedure 39-3 **Administering Oxygen Therapy**	Able to Perform	Able to Perform with Assistance	Unable to Perform	Initials and Date
Assessment				
1. Determine client history and acute and chronic health problems. *Comments:*	☐	☐	☐	
2. Assess the client's baseline respiratory signs. *Comments:*	☐	☐	☐	
3. Check the extremities and mucous membranes for color. *Comments:*	☐	☐	☐	
4. Review arterial blood gas (ABG) and pulse oximetry results. *Comments:*	☐	☐	☐	
5. Note lung sounds for rales and rhonchi. *Comments:*	☐	☐	☐	
6. Assess the skin in places where tubing or equipment contacts the skin. *Comments:*	☐	☐	☐	
Planning/Expected Outcomes				
1. Oxygen levels will return to normal in blood and tissues. *Comments:*	☐	☐	☐	
2. Respiratory rate, pattern, and depth will be within the normal range. *Comments:*	☐	☐	☐	
3. The client will not develop any skin breakdown. *Comments:*	☐	☐	☐	
4. Breathing efficiency and activity tolerance will be increased. *Comments:*	☐	☐	☐	

continued on the following page

continued from the previous page

Procedure 39-3	Able to Perform	Able to Perform with Assistance	Unable to Perform	Initials and Date
5. The client will understand the rationale for the therapy. *Comments:*	☐	☐	☐	

Implementation

Nasal Cannula

	Able to Perform	Able to Perform with Assistance	Unable to Perform	Initials and Date
1. Wash hands. *Comments:*	☐	☐	☐	
2. Verify the written order. *Comments:*	☐	☐	☐	
3. Explain procedure and hazards to the client. *Comments:*	☐	☐	☐	
4. Fill humidifier to fill line with distilled water and close container. *Comments:*	☐	☐	☐	
5. Attach humidifier to oxygen flow meter. *Comments:*	☐	☐	☐	
6. Insert humidifier and flow meter into oxygen source. *Comments:*	☐	☐	☐	
7. Attach the oxygen tubing and nasal cannula to the flow meter and turn it on to the prescribed flow rate (1–5 L/m). *Comments:*	☐	☐	☐	
8. Check for bubbling in the humidifier. *Comments:*	☐	☐	☐	
9. Place the nasal prongs in the client's nostrils, and secure the cannula over the client's ears. *Comments:*	☐	☐	☐	
10. Check for proper flow rate every 4 hours. *Comments:*	☐	☐	☐	
11. Assess client nostrils every 8 hours. *Comments:*	☐	☐	☐	

continued from the previous page

Procedure 39-3	Able to Perform	Able to Perform with Assistance	Unable to Perform	Initials and Date
12. Monitor vital signs, oxygen saturation, and client condition every 4 to 8 hours. *Comments:*	☐	☐	☐	
13. Wean clients from oxygen as soon as possible using standard protocols. *Comments:*	☐	☐	☐	
Mask 14. Wash hands. *Comments:*	☐	☐	☐	
15. Repeat steps 2 through 6. *Comments:*	☐	☐	☐	
16. Attach appropriately sized mask or face tent to oxygen tubing and turn on flow meter to prescribed flow rate. *Comments:*	☐	☐	☐	
17. Check for bubbling in the humidifier. *Comments:*	☐	☐	☐	
18. Place the mask or tent on the client's face and fasten snugly with elastic band. *Comments:*	☐	☐	☐	
19. Check for proper flow rate every 4 hours. *Comments:*	☐	☐	☐	
20. Ensure that the ports of the Venturi mask are not blocked. *Comments:*	☐	☐	☐	
21. Assess client's skin for pressure areas and pad as needed. *Comments:*	☐	☐	☐	
22. Wean client to nasal cannula and then off oxygen per protocol. *Comments:*	☐	☐	☐	

     continued on the following page

continued from the previous page

Procedure 39-3	Able to Perform	Able to Perform with Assistance	Unable to Perform	Initials and Date
Oxygen via an Artificial Airway				
23. Wash hands. *Comments:*	☐	☐	☐	
24. Verify the written order. *Comments:*	☐	☐	☐	
25. Fill the humidifier with water and close the container. *Comments:*	☐	☐	☐	
26. Attach humidifier and warmer to the oxygen flow meter. *Comments:*	☐	☐	☐	
27. Attach wide-bore oxygen tubing and T-tube adapter or tracheostomy mask to the flow meter. Initiate oxygen at the prescribed rate. *Comments:*	☐	☐	☐	
28. Check for bubbling in the humidifier and a fine mist from the adapter. *Comments:*	☐	☐	☐	
29. Attach the T-piece to the client's artificial airway or place the mask over the client's airway. *Comments:*	☐	☐	☐	
30. Position tubing so that it is not pulling client's airway. *Comments:*	☐	☐	☐	
31. Check for proper flow rate and patency of the system every 1 to 2 hours. Suction as needed to maintain a patent airway. *Comments:*	☐	☐	☐	
32. Monitor for signs and symptoms of hypoxia every 2 hours. Monitor breath sounds and tube position every 4 hours. *Comments:*	☐	☐	☐	
33. Wean client from therapy as ordered by qualified practitioner. *Comments:*	☐	☐	☐	

_____   _____

Faculty Signature   Date

Checklist for Procedure 39-4   Performing the Heimlich Maneuver

Name _____ Date _____

School _____

Instructor _____

Course _____

Procedure 39-4 Performing the Heimlich Maneuver	Able to Perform	Able to Perform with Assistance	Unable to Perform	Initials and Date
Assessment				
1. Assess air exchange. *Comments:*	☐	☐	☐	
2. Establish airway obstruction. *Comments:*	☐	☐	☐	
3. Differentiate between infection and airway obstruction. *Comments:*	☐	☐	☐	
Planning/Expected Outcomes				
1. The client's clinical status will improve. *Comments:*	☐	☐	☐	
2. The client's gas exchange will improve. *Comments:*	☐	☐	☐	
3. The client will experience minimal discomfort during airway clearance. *Comments:*	☐	☐	☐	
4. The client will not experience complications. *Comments:*	☐	☐	☐	
Implementation				
Foreign Body Obstruction—All Clients 1. Assess airway for complete or partial blockage. *Comments:*	☐	☐	☐	
2. Activate emergency response assistance. *Comments:*	☐	☐	☐	

    continued on the following page

continued from the previous page

Procedure 39-4	Able to Perform	Able to Perform with Assistance	Unable to Perform	Initials and Date
Conscious Adult Client—Sitting or Standing (Heimlich Maneuver)				
3. Stand behind the client. *Comments:*	☐	☐	☐	
4. Wrap your arms around the client's waist. *Comments:*	☐	☐	☐	
5. Make a fist with one hand and grasp it with your other hand, placing the thumb side of the fist against the client's abdomen. *Comments:*	☐	☐	☐	
6. Perform a quick upward thrust into the client's abdomen. *Comments:*	☐	☐	☐	
7. Repeat this process six to ten times until the client either expels the foreign body or loses consciousness. *Comments:*	☐	☐	☐	
Adult Client Who Is or Becomes Unconscious				
8. Repeat steps 1 and 2. *Comments:*	☐	☐	☐	
9. With the client supine, kneel astride the client's abdomen. *Comments:*	☐	☐	☐	
10. Place the heel of one hand below the xiphoid process and above the navel. Place the second hand on top of the first hand. *Comments:*	☐	☐	☐	
11. Perform a quick upward thrust into the diaphragm, repeating six to ten times. *Comments:*	☐	☐	☐	
12. Perform a finger sweep. *Comments:*	☐	☐	☐	
13. Open the client's airway and attempt ventilation. *Comments:*	☐	☐	☐	

Procedure 39-4	Able to Perform	Able to Perform with Assistance	Unable to Perform	Initials and Date
14. Continue sequence of Heimlich maneuver, finger sweep, and rescue breathing as long as necessary. *Comments:*	☐	☐	☐	
Conscious Adult Sitting or Standing—Chest Thrusts 15. Repeat steps 1 and 2. *Comments:*	☐	☐	☐	
16. Stand behind the client and encircle the chest with arms under the axilla. *Comments:*	☐	☐	☐	
17. Make a fist and place the thumb side of the fist on the middle of the client's sternum and grasp the fist with the second hand. *Comments:*	☐	☐	☐	
18. Perform backward thrusts until the client either becomes unconscious or the foreign body is expelled. *Comments:*	☐	☐	☐	
Unconscious Adult—Chest Thrusts 19. Repeat steps 1 and 2. *Comments:*	☐	☐	☐	
20. Place client supine and kneel at the client's side. *Comments:*	☐	☐	☐	
21. Place the heel of one hand on the lower half of the sternum. *Comments:*	☐	☐	☐	
22. Perform each thrust in a slow, separate, and distinct manner. *Comments:*	☐	☐	☐	
23. Follow steps 9 through 12 for the adult Heimlich maneuver, unconscious client. *Comments:*	☐	☐	☐	

continued on the following page

continued from the previous page

Procedure 39-4	Able to Perform	Able to Perform with Assistance	Unable to Perform	Initials and Date
Airway Obstruction—Infants and Small Children 24. Differentiate between infection and airway obstruction. *Comments:*	☐	☐	☐	
Infant Airway Obstruction 25. Straddle infant over forearm in the prone position with the head lower than the trunk. Support the infant's head in the open palm of the hand. *Comments:*	☐	☐	☐	
26. Deliver four back blows between the infant's shoulder blades. *Comments:*	☐	☐	☐	
27. Keeping the infant's head down, turn the infant over. *Comments:*	☐	☐	☐	
28. Deliver four thrusts as in infant external cardiac compressions. *Comments:*	☐	☐	☐	
29. Assess for a foreign body in an unconscious infant. Utilize the finger sweep only if a foreign body is visualized. *Comments:*	☐	☐	☐	
30. Open airway and assess for respiration. If respirations are absent, attempt rescue breathing. *Comments:*	☐	☐	☐	
31. Repeat the entire sequence as long as necessary. *Comments:*	☐	☐	☐	
Small Child—Airway Obstruction (Conscious, Standing or Sitting) 32. Assess air exchange, and encourage coughing and breathing. *Comments:*	☐	☐	☐	

Procedure 39-4	Able to Perform	Able to Perform with Assistance	Unable to Perform	Initials and Date
33. If the child has poor air exchange, initiate the following steps: • Stand behind the child with your arms wrapped around the waist and administer six to ten subdiaphragmatic abdominal thrusts. • Continue until foreign object is expelled or the child becomes unconscious. *Comments:*	☐	☐	☐	
Small Child—Airway Obstruction (Conscious or Unconscious, Lying) 34. Position the child supine and kneel at the child's feet. Gently deliver six to ten subdiaphragmatic abdominal thrusts. *Comments:*	☐	☐	☐	
35. Open airway. Perform a finger sweep only if a foreign body is visualized. *Comments:*	☐	☐	☐	
36. If breathing is absent, begin rescue breathing. *Comments:*	☐	☐	☐	
37. Repeat this sequence as long as necessary. *Comments:*	☐	☐	☐	
38. Wash hands. *Comments:*	☐	☐	☐	

_____

Faculty Signature

Date

Checklist for Procedure 39-5   Administering Cardiopulmonary Resuscitation (CPR)

Name _____ Date _____

School _____

Instructor _____

Course _____

Procedure 39-5 Administering Cardiopulmonary Resuscitation (CPR)	Able to Perform	Able to Perform with Assistance	Unable to Perform	Initials and Date
Assessment				
1. Assess responsiveness and level of consciousness. *Comments:*	☐	☐	☐	
2. Assess the amount and abilities of any available assistance. *Comments:*	☐	☐	☐	
3. Assess the client's position. *Comments:*	☐	☐	☐	
4. Assess respiratory status. *Comments:*	☐	☐	☐	
5. Assess circulatory status. *Comments:*	☐	☐	☐	
Planning/Expected Outcomes				
1. Client will experience improved clinical status. *Comments:*	☐	☐	☐	
2. Client does not experience negative sequela related to hypoxic event. *Comments:*	☐	☐	☐	
3. Client does not have damage inflicted secondary to CPR. *Comments:*	☐	☐	☐	
4. Cardiopulmonary resuscitation was terminated appropriately. *Comments:*	☐	☐	☐	
Implementation				
CPR: One Rescuer—Adult, Adolescent				
1. Assess responsiveness. *Comments:*	☐	☐	☐	

    continued on the following page

continued from the previous page

Procedure 39-5	Able to Perform	Able to Perform with Assistance	Unable to Perform	Initials and Date
2. Activate emergency medical system. *Comments:*	☐	☐	☐	
3. Position client in a supine position on a hard, flat surface. *Comments:*	☐	☐	☐	
4. Apply appropriate body substance isolation items, if available. *Comments:*	☐	☐	☐	
5. Position self. *Comments:*	☐	☐	☐	
6. Open airway. *Comments:*	☐	☐	☐	
7. Assess for respirations. *Comments:*	☐	☐	☐	
8. If respirations are absent: • Occlude nostrils with the thumb and index finger. • Form a seal over the client's mouth with your mouth or the appropriate device. Give two full breaths. • Mouth-to-nose ventilation may be used. • In an agency setting, use appropriate Ambu bag to provide ventilatory support. *Comments:*	☐	☐	☐	
9. Assess for the rise and fall of the chest: • If present, continue to step 10. • If absent, assess for airway obstruction. *Comments:*	☐	☐	☐	
10. Palpate the carotid pulse: • If present, continue rescue breathing. • If absent, begin cardiac compressions. *Comments:*	☐	☐	☐	
11. Cardiac compressions: • Maintain a position on knees parallel to sternum. • Position the hands for compressions. • Extend or interlace fingers. • Keep arms straight and lock elbows. • Compress at the age-appropriate rate. • Ventilate client as described in step 8. *Comments:*	☐	☐	☐	

Procedure 39-5	Able to Perform	Able to Perform with Assistance	Unable to Perform	Initials and Date
12. Maintain the appropriate compression rate, interjecting ventilation after every 15 compressions. *Comments:*	☐	☐	☐	
13. Reassess the client after four cycles. *Comments:*	☐	☐	☐	
CPR: Two Rescuers—Adult, Adolescent 14. Follow steps 1 through 13 with the following changes: • Rescuers are positioned on opposite sides of the client. • The rescuer at the trunk performs cardiac compressions and maintains the verbal count. This is rescuer 1. • The rescuer positioned at the head monitors respirations, assesses pulse, establishes an airway, and performs rescue breathing. This is rescuer 2. • The compression-to-ventilation rate changes to 5:1. • Rescuer 2 palpates the carotid pulse throughout the first full minute. • When either rescuer calls for a change, he completes his portion of the cycle and the rescuers switch positions. • The client's status is reassessed after each change. If cardiac arrest persists, CPR is continued. *Comments:*	☐	☐	☐	
CPR: One Rescuer—Child (1–7 years) 15. Follow steps 1 through 7. *Comments:*	☐	☐	☐	
16. If respirations are absent, begin rescue breathing. *Comments:*	☐	☐	☐	
17. Palpate the carotid pulse. • If present, continue ventilation. • If absent, begin cardiac compressions. *Comments:*	☐	☐	☐	
18. Cardiac compressions (child 1–7 years): • Maintain a position on knees parallel to child's sternum. • Place a small towel under the child's shoulders. • Place the heel of one hand one finger-breadth below the level of the nipple line for chest compressions. • At the end of every fifth compression, administer a ventilation. • Reevaluate child after 10 cycles. *Comments:*	☐	☐	☐	

continued on the following page

continued from the previous page

Procedure 39-5	Able to Perform	Able to Perform with Assistance	Unable to Perform	Initials and Date
CPR: One Rescuer—Infant (1–12 months) 19. Follow steps 1 through 7. *Comments:*	☐	☐	☐	
20. If respirations are absent, begin rescue breathing. *Comments:*	☐	☐	☐	
21. Assess circulatory status using the brachial pulse. • If a pulse is palpated, continue rescue breathing. • If a pulse is absent, begin cardiac compressions. *Comments:*	☐	☐	☐	
22. Cardiac compressions (infant 1–12 months): • Maintain a position parallel to the infant. • Place a small towel under the infant's shoulders/neck. • Place two fingers one finger-breadth below the level of the nipple line for chest compressions in an infant. • Reevaluate infant after 10 cycles. *Comments:*	☐	☐	☐	
CPR: Two Rescuers—Child (1–7 years) and Infant (1–12 months) 23. Follow step 14, except: • Utilize the child or infant procedure for chest compressions. • Change the ratio of compressions to ventilation to 3:1. • Deliver the ventilation on the upstroke of the third compression. *Comments:*	☐	☐	☐	
CPR: Neonate or Premature Infant 24. Follow the infant guidelines except: • Encircle the chest with both hands. • Position thumbs over the midsternum. • Compress the midsternum with both thumbs. *Comments:*	☐	☐	☐	

_____   _____

Faculty Signature   Date